POST-TRAUMATIC FIBROMYALGIA

A MEDICAL PERSPECTIVE

BY

MARK J. PELLEGRINO, M.D.

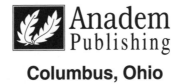
Anadem
Publishing

Columbus, Ohio

POST-TRAUMATIC FIBROMYALGIA
A MEDICAL PERSPECTIVE

3620 North High Street
Columbus, Ohio 43214
614 • 262 • 2539
800 • 633 • 0055

The material in *Post-Traumatic Fibromyalgia* is presented for informational purposes only. It is not meant to be a substitute for proper medical care by your doctor. You need to consult with your doctor for diagnosis and treatment.

The material is not meant to take the place of consultation with an attorney or other qualified professional.

ISBN 0-9646891-8-9

Table of Contents

Fibromyalgia is a common condition causing painful muscles. In recent years, increased awareness of what previously was a mysterious and controversial condition has made fibromyalgia a well-recognized and legitimate syndrome. Health care professionals of all specialties are involved in treating fibromyalgia patients.

Fibromyalgia frequently occurs following trauma. The medical, legal and work costs for post-traumatic fibromyalgia are estimated to be billions of dollars a year.

I have fibromyalgia and understand how this condition causes persistent pain affecting one's everyday life. As a physiatrist (specialist in physical medicine and rehabilitation), I have diagnosed and treated thousands of patients with fibromyalgia. Conducting research projects, attending international symposiums, and reading the latest medical literature have contributed greatly to my base of knowledge, but I have also learned much from the many patients with fibromyalgia that I treat in my private practice. I have the unique opportunity of bridging both my personal and professional interests in this condition.

Over the years, I have gained a lot of experience with patients who have fibromyalgia related to trauma, i.e. post-traumatic fibromyalgia. The purpose of this book is to enhance one's awareness of post-traumatic fibromyalgia from a medical perspective based on my background and experiences combined with the current scientific knowledge.

For those just beginning to learn about fibromyalgia, I have included some of the basic introductory material that was first presented in *Fibromyalgia: Managing the Pain*. Those desiring more information about primary fibromyalgia are urged to read *Fibromyalgia: Managing the Pain* and *The Fibromyalgia Survivor*. (For more information, call Anadem Publishing, 800-633-0055.)

This book is for informational purposes only. It is not meant to be a substitute for proper medical care or legal advice.

1

Fibromyalgia: The Basics

Fibromyalgia is a syndrome of chronic muscle pain that is recognized as a distinct medical condition with characteristic findings. The pain involves many muscles, tendons, ligaments, bursa, and joints. Distinct areas of tenderness in specific locations called "tender points" are characteristic findings. According to the American College of Rheumatology criteria, at least 11 of 18 specific body locations must have painful tender points in order to diagnose generalized fibromyalgia. Regional fibromyalgia and myofascial pain syndrome can occur with fewer than 11 tender points.

The muscle pain fluctuates and is often aggravated by various physical, environmental and emotional factors. In addition to pain, fibromyalgia causes stiffness, fatigue, numbness, feeling of weakness, swelling, cold intolerance, poor sleep and dry eyes, as well as other symptoms. Various conditions have been linked to fibromyalgia, including tension and migraine headaches, chest pain, mitral valve prolapse, irritable bowel syndrome, TMJ dysfunction, irritable bladder, depression and chronic fatigue syndrome.

Fibromyalgia is diagnosed more frequently in women than in men, occurring in about 2 - 5% of the population. Children can also have fibromyalgia, although the condition usually causes symptoms that begin between ages 25 and 45. For many patients, the symptoms may be present for years even though the diagnosis may not be made until past age 50.

Fibromyalgia can be classified into different types.

TABLE 1: TYPES OF FIBROMYALGIA

Primary fibromyalgia	This is the most common type and occurs in the absence of any underlying rheumatologic disease such as rheumatoid arthritis or lupus. Usually at least 11 of 18 designated tender points are positive in this type. Genetics are felt to play a major role.
Concomitant fibromyalgia	This is thought to occur along with another condition such as osteoarthritis or scoliosis, with no clear relationship.
Secondary (or reactive) fibromyalgia	This category has two types: a. Fibromyalgia that occurs in the presence of an underlying disease such as rheumatoid arthritis, lupus, hypothyroidism or cancer. This type is usually generalized, with at least 11 of 18 designated tender points. Even though fibromyalgia symptoms may be more severe than the underlying disease symptoms, the underlying disease is considered the cause of the fibromyalgia and both conditions need to be treated. b. Post-traumatic fibromyalgia is a special category of secondary fibromyalgia commonly seen following a trauma such as a motor vehicle accident or work injury. This particular type of fibromyalgia will be emphasized in this book.
Regional Fibromyalgia	This more localized form of fibromyalgia has fewer than 11 of 18 positive tender points.

Myofascial pain syndrome is also a common condition causing muscle pain and may be a regional or localized form of fibromyalgia (although some doctors consider it to be a separate entity altogether). In myofascial pain syndrome, there exist painful tender points that are more localized, and trigger points which, when pressed on, cause referred pain or numbness to a different area. In generalized and regional fibromyalgia, both tender and trigger points are present.

> *Since the tender point abnormalities seen in myofascial pain syndrome are identical to the ones in fibromyalgia, I believe myofascial pain syndrome is the same as regional fibromyalgia. Both may eventually develop into generalized fibromyalgia.*

Associated conditions such as irritable bowel syndrome, irritable bladder and depression are usually not seen with myofascial pain syndrome as they are with generalized fibromyalgia, but they can occur. Since the tender point abnormalities seen in myofascial pain syndrome are identical to the ones in fibromyalgia, I believe myofascial pain syndrome is the same as regional fibromyalgia. Both are frequently caused by muscle trauma, and both may eventually develop into generalized fibromyalgia.

The exact cause of fibromyalgia is unknown, but ongoing research continues to shed light on this syndrome. A variety of factors are considered to be important in causing fibromyalgia: genetics, trauma, altered neurologic mechanisms, muscle physiology problems, infectious disorders, abnormal sleep patterns, structural muscle changes, neurotransmitter abnormalities, endocrine abnormalities, immune disorders and allergic factors. Some of the more recent research has focused on growth hormone abnormalities, abnormal biochemical mechanisms involving various enzyme systems, brain, hypothalamus and neurologic dysfunctions, and altered oxygen/energy mechanisms.

After a person is diagnosed with fibromyalgia syndrome, a multidisciplinary treatment approach often helps. Education on this condition should emphasize that fibromyalgia is not a deadly or contagious disease and that a person can learn to successfully live with this condition. Various medications including muscle relaxants, sleep modifiers, antidepressants and pain relievers can be helpful. Trigger point injections and "spray and stretch" can also help. Physical therapies, massage, manipulation, psychological treatment, occupational therapy and other treatments can decrease pain and improve one's ability to cope with this condition. A key strategy is learning a home program that works.

Fibromyalgia is a chronic and permanent condition for which there is no cure. Physicians of all specialties are learning more about fibromyalgia and are becoming better at diagnosing and treating this condition. The challenge is not only to fully understand fibromyalgia, but also to minimize its effect on the individual and the community until a cure is found.

2

Many physicians continue to describe fibromyalgia as a controversial condition. However, to those of us who are well informed, there is no question at all about the existence of this condition. Fibromyalgia is indeed a real syndrome with characteristic findings.

Part of the controversy stems from the fact that fibromyalgia was originally described as "fibrositis" as a cause of low back pain. Medical investigators in the early 1900s reported that they had seen inflamed areas of fibrous tissue or fascia that surrounds muscles and binds them together, when this area was observed under a microscope. Hence the name "fibrositis," which implied that the cause of the pain was a fibrous tissue inflammation ("fibro" = fibrous tissue, "itis" = inflammation).

With the advent of more sophisticated microscopes and carefully designed research studies, medical investigators observed that there was no actual inflammation in the muscles or connective tissues of these patients. Because the original opinion that an inflammation existed was wrong, many doctors falsely concluded that fibrositis was therefore not even a legitimate condition, and that the patient's symptoms were "all in the head." In fact, many physicians used the term "psychogenic rheumatism" to describe fibrositis. For many years fibrositis was considered a "wastebasket diagnosis" of patients with chronic pain for which all the tests were normal and no disease was found. Different names were used: fibrositis, fibromyositis, tension myalgia, myofascial pain syndrome and more. All described the same syndrome of chronic muscle pain.

In the late 1960s and early 1970s, more articles appeared describing fibrositis (now called fibromyalgia) in the journals of *Physical Medicine and Rehabilitation* and *Rheumatology*. Dr. Travell researched trigger points and referred pain called myofascial pain. Dr. Moldofsky performed sleep studies and found characteristic stage 4 sleep abnormalities in individuals with fibromyalgia. Dr. Johnson wrote about treatments for fibrositis.

In 1981, Dr. Yunus described criteria which were used as a standard to objectively diagnose patients with fibrositis. A virtual explosion of research has occurred since then, and in 1987, Dr. Goldenberg published an important overview article on fibromyalgia in the most widely read scientific journal, the *Journal of the American Medical Association* (JAMA). This article and the accompanying editorial by Dr. Bennett validated the existence of fibromyalgia as a legitimate syndrome recognized by the American Medical Association. Around this time, the name "fibromyalgia" was felt to be the best name as it described pain ("algia") in fibrous ("fibro") and muscle ("mya") tissues.

In 1989, investigators worldwide convened in Minneapolis for the First International Myofascial Pain and Fibromyalgia Symposium to present research and share knowledge. In 1990, a multicenter study organized by Dr. Wolfe determined diagnostic criteria using tender points as the key distinguishing physical findings in fibromyalgia. This landmark study has been considered the "gold standard" for diagnosing fibromyalgia.

Further studies on the neurotransmitters and hormones have yielded important clues about the pathology of fibromyalgia. Substance P has been found to be elevated, serotonin is low, growth hormone and cortisol levels are low. Muscle energy molecules called ATP are depleted. Numerous other abnormalities are present in fibromyalgia. (For more in-depth information about neurotransmitters and hormones, see Chapter 7, Diagnostic Testing in Post-Traumatic Fibromyalgia.)

> *Fibromyalgia has been discussed in hundreds of articles in numerous scientific journals and consumer magazines involving all types of medical professionals.*

In 1992, the Second International Myofascial Pain and Fibromyalgia Symposium was held in Copenhagen, Denmark, attracting over 500 medical professionals throughout the world interested in fibromyalgia. In the summer of 1995, investigators and healthcare professionals worldwide convened in San Antonio, Texas, for the Third World Congress on Myofascial Pain and Fibromyalgia with the emphasis on the pathophysiologic mechanisms of pain. Research and advocacy organizations have developed, and more and more research money and grants are being funneled into fibromyalgia to further study this disorder.

Fibromyalgia has been discussed in hundreds of articles in numerous scientific journals and consumer magazines involving all types of medical professionals. Support groups and newsletters promoting public awareness and understanding of this condition have multiplied.

The courts have recognized fibromyalgia as a legitimate condition. Fibromyalgia is listed as a diagnosis in the Universal CPT codings of medical diagnoses. It is virtually impossible to ignore the expanse of literature and research on this condition, and although this condition may have many mysteries that need to be solved, it is not at all controversial in its existence.

> *It is virtually impossible to ignore the expanse of literature and research on this condition, and although this condition may have many mysteries that need to be solved, it is not at all controversial in its existence.*

In spite of this overwhelming evidence, some physicians will try to state that fibromyalgia's existence is controversial. It is my opinion that a well-informed physician would never make such a statement as the scientific evidence is indeed overwhelming. It has been my experience that physicians who do not recognize fibromyalgia or try to state that it is controversial are not knowledgeable in the diagnosis of fibromyalgia or experienced in the art of palpating painful muscles and documenting the presence of tender points.

Part of the problem has been the lack of education on fibromyalgia at the medical school and residency level. As we have learned more about this condition in the past decade, medical schools and residencies have assimilated fibromyalgia and its treatment into the overall curriculum. Consequently more and more physicians who have just completed their training are knowledgeable about fibromyalgia and its treatment. Physicians who do not have the benefit of this knowledge and have not read the scientific literature on this condition may deny the existence of fibromyalgia.

Medicine is an ever-evolving science. It is the responsibility of every physician to continue the learning process beyond medical school and residency program. Just because we have not learned about a particular condition, or treated it before, does not mean that it does not exist. Regardless of the individual's background or credentials, if a physician tries to state an "expert opinion" that fibromyalgia does not exist, he or she is not in compliance with the current scientific standard of knowledge. A knowledgeable attorney should be able to portray this doctor's so called "expert testimony" as unreliable testimony not consistent with factual scientific knowledge.

> *If a physician tries to state an "expert opinion" that fibromyalgia does not exist, he or she is not in compliance with the current scientific standard of knowledge. A knowledgeable attorney can portray this doctor's testimony as unreliable and not consistent with factual scientific knowledge.*

Fibromyalgia is a unique syndrome that is diagnosed and treated by all types of medical professionals. Legal and government agencies recognize this condition as a "legitimate" one. We will explore post-traumatic fibromyalgia in detail in the remainder of this book.

3

Post-Traumatic Fibromyalgia Overview

Post-traumatic fibromyalgia is a type of fibromyalgia that is caused by trauma. As discussed in Chapter 1, I have classified post-traumatic fibromyalgia as a type of secondary (or reactive) fibromyalgia. This classification is given because the trauma directly causes soft tissue changes that lead to the clinical syndrome of fibromyalgia.

Some physicians feel that post-traumatic fibromyalgia should be classified as a form of primary fibromyalgia. Dr. Waylonis published a study in the *American Journal of Physical Medicine and Rehabilitation* (1994), in which his observations supported the hypothesis that primary fibromyalgia and post-traumatic fibromyalgia actually represent a single condition and that separation into different types is artificial.

A key historical difference, however, is that individuals with post-traumatic fibromyalgia report a trauma at the onset of their painful condition, whereas individuals with primary fibromyalgia do not. The basis on which classification of post-traumatic fibromyalgia should be given is purely academic and not clinically significant as the majority of physicians who treat fibromyalgia recognize that trauma can be a precipitating factor in the development of painful fibromyalgia syndrome. Whether post-traumatic fibromyalgia is a special classification of primary fibromyalgia or a subset of sec-

ondary fibromyalgia is not to be deemed a controversy in fibromyalgia. I favor the secondary fibromyalgia classification.

Trauma to the muscle, simply defined, is a physical injury to the muscle causing
pathological changes. There are
two types of trauma that may
lead to post-traumatic fibromyalgia, macroscopic and microscopic.

> *An injury can still be catego-
> rized as macroscopic trauma
> even if there is no visible
> swelling, hemorrhage or other
> muscle changes.*

Macroscopic trauma is caused
by a sudden forceful injury to the
muscle. The traumatic forces occur over a brief
period of time, often milliseconds, that are usually
a one-time insult. Such a macroscopic trauma could
occur during a whiplash injury, or as the result of a
blunt injury from a fall, being struck by an object,
or a back sprain from sudden lifting of a heavy
object. All of these examples are considered "obvious" traumas.

Microscopic trauma occurs by a different mechanism. It represents a more subtle, low-grade type
of trauma that occurs over time from cumulative
and repetitive actions on the muscles. There is no
one "obvious" trauma, but a series of low-grade
muscle insults that, over time, lead to pathological
changes. Although individuals can often recall the
exact moment of injury in macroscopic trauma, they
usually will not remember any obvious single injury in microscopic trauma.

Examples of microscopic trauma include shoulder
strain in an assembly-line worker who has done a
lot of reaching and pushing for several years, wrist
strains in a secretary who spends hours a day typing on a computer keyboard, and neck strain in a
school bus driver who looks in the overhead mirror
to monitor the activities on the inside of the bus.

Macroscopic and microscopic traumas describe the mechanism of trauma, but not the actual changes occurring at a pathological level. Regardless of the trauma type, pathologic changes that occur include swelling or edema, and hemorrhage due to disruption and tears of the muscle fibers. These changes are usually detected on a microscopic level. Many times there is a swelling or hemorrhage which is visible to the eye in macroscopic trauma, but not always. An injury can still be categorized as macroscopic trauma even if there is no visible swelling, hemorrhage or other muscle changes.

> *Post-traumatic fibromyalgia does not develop immediately after the injury. It takes time for this condition to evolve and fully develop the characteristic painful tender points in distinct locations.*

While muscle trauma as described causes pathological changes in the muscles, not all trauma leads to post-traumatic fibromyalgia. Traumas can cause:

- Strains (from injury to the muscle due to over-stretching or overexertion)
- Sprains (muscle and ligament injury where fiber disruption occurs)
- Avulsions (the tearing away of part of a muscle or ligament)
- Other types of acute injuries.

Post-traumatic fibromyalgia does not develop immediately after the injury. It takes time for this condition to evolve and fully develop the characteristic painful tender points in distinct locations. The initial trauma causes soft-tissue pathologic changes in which the damage is done on a microscopic level. The body tries to heal the injury and begins a chain of events that lead to development of painful tender points and ultimately, the full expression of post-traumatic fibromyalgia. This process takes several months to develop, and once it develops it is permanent.

Post-traumatic fibromyalgia usually causes pain in tender points localized to the region of the injury. The regions injured may include only the neck and shoulders, but the injury may be more expansive and involve the entire back. If the pain is localized rather than generalized in distribution, the individual may not develop 11 of 18 tender points to meet the criteria for generalized fibromyalgia syndrome set by the American College of Rheumatology. As I have indicated, however, this does not mean the person does not have fibromyalgia; rather, the person has a regional form of post-traumatic fibromyalgia.

> *If the pain is more localized in distribution, the individual may not develop 11 of 18 tender points to meet the criteria for generalized fibromyalgia syndrome. This does not mean the person does not have fibromyalgia; rather, the person has a regional form of post-traumatic fibromyalgia.*

Doctors who treat fibromyalgia observe that patients with regional post-traumatic fibromyalgia may develop more generalization of their pain over time. For example, a person who had a whiplash injury and was bothered mainly by neck and shoulder pain which led to typical painful tender points and a diagnosis of regional post-traumatic fibromyalgia, may start developing low-back pain or pain in other areas that were never injured by the accident. Similarly, a factory worker who lifted a box and experienced low back strain and ultimately had regional post-traumatic fibromyalgia may, over time, start experiencing neck and shoulder pain. Upon examination by a doctor, these persons may demonstrate generalized painful tender points that meet these criteria (at least 11 of 18 painful tender points) for generalized fibromyalgia. This "spreading" of fibromyalgia will be discussed in a later chapter.

If an individual has persistent pain and painful tender points at least six months following a trauma, post-traumatic fibromyalgia is present. Furthermore, the probability is high that the post-traumatic fibromyalgia and its associated tender points will continue to persist indefinitely and be a chronic and permanent condition.

Physical trauma has been cited by the majority of patients as the cause of their myofascial pain syndrome when the onset of pain was abrupt.

There are various studies investigating post-traumatic fibromyalgia in the medical literature. Dr. Romano, in 1990, wrote an article describing patients with post-traumatic fibromyalgia continuing to require treatment for their condition even years after settlement of litigation. In 1992, Dr. Greenfield published a paper describing reactive fibromyalgia syndrome in which patients with fibromyalgia commonly reported trauma as a precipitating event.

Dr. Goldenberg, one of the foremost authorities on fibromyalgia, has reported that 55% to 60% of his fibromyalgia patients attribute the onset of their fibromyalgia symptoms to a traumatic or infectious event. Dr. Waylonis published a paper entitled "Post Traumatic Fibromyalgia, A Long-Term Follow-Up" in 1994 that describes a follow-up study of 176 individuals with a diagnosis of post-traumatic fibromyalgia.

Numerous studies by various authors including Dr. Simons have described myofascial pain syndrome with associated tender and trigger points that commonly develop following trauma. Localized or regional myofascial pain syndrome can become more generalized over time. Physical trauma has been cited by the majority of patients as the cause of their myofascial pain syndrome when the onset of pain was abrupt.

FIGURE 1: TYPES OF TRAUMA LEADING TO POST-TRAUMATIC FIBROMYALGIA

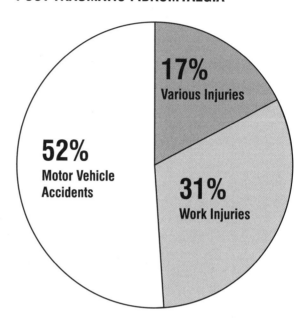

Studies written earlier than 1990 have investigated persistent pain following soft-tissue injuries including a broader category of "chronic soft tissue pain syndrome." However, these earlier studies did not distinguish or separate out post-traumatic fibromyalgia because the definitive criteria had not yet been established. In the past few years, there has been an increased interest by physicians, attorneys, insurance companies, disability bureaus and workers' compensation bureaus on post-traumatic fibromyalgia and long-term outcomes.

In my own private practice, I have analyzed patients with a diagnosis of fibromyalgia. From 1990 to 1995, 2000 records of fibromyalgia patients were reviewed. Of those, 65% reported the onset of their symptoms of fibromyalgia after a traumatic event. Of this group of post-traumatic fibromyalgia patients, 52% of them were involved in motor vehicle accidents, 31% had work injuries, and the remaining 17% had another type of trauma. In this other trauma category, various injuries included:

- Sports injuries
- Recreational injuries
- Fractures
- Surgical procedures
- Head injuries
- Pregnancy

Of the post-traumatic patients involved in motor vehicle accidents, whiplash injury was the most common type of trauma. This injury will be discussed in Chapter 4. The literature and individual practitioners' experiences are revealing that many patients seen with fibromyalgia have had some type of trauma that caused their conditions. Doctors who treat large numbers of fibromyalgia patients report that the majority have trauma-related or post-traumatic fibromyalgia.

4

The Whiplash Injury

The whiplash injury is one of the most common injuries sustained during a motor vehicle accident. This injury can occur with a rear-end collision, a side collision or a head-on collision. Whiplash injury is one of the most common causes of post-traumatic fibromyalgia.

What happens during a rear-end collision? An individual sitting in a stopped car that is suddenly rear-ended will be exposed to a rapid-fire chain of events involving the head and neck. The impact causes the body (which acts as part of the car) to

FIGURE 2: WHIPLASH INJURY

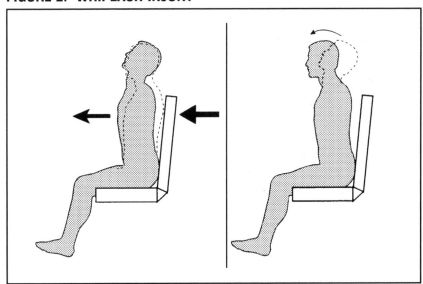

abruptly move forward. The head, however, stays in its same position briefly due to inertia. While the rest of the body is moving forward, the head (acting as an independent 10-pound object) is staying in the same position but, relative to the body, is abruptly jerking backwards or hyperextending.

Headrests don't stop neck injuries when a car is rear-ended; 97% of new cars have headrests that cannot be positioned properly or do not stay in place during a crash, offering little protection against neck injuries.

This sudden movement occurs upon unprepared cervical spine ligaments and muscles. This sudden hyperextension activates protective stretch reflexes in the front muscles of the neck which cause the head to jerk forward (or hyperflex) to catch up with the rest of the body. These jerking backward (hyperextension) and forward (hyperflexion) movements are the "whiplash" effects; hence, the whiplash injury.

A head-on collision would cause the opposite reaction, with the neck violently flexing forward first, followed by a rebound extension or jerking backward effect. A side collision will cause side or lateral movements of the head combined with flexion and extension. A side-front collision will cause lateral/flexion movements followed by rebound opposite lateral/extension movements, whereas a side-rear collision will cause the reverse order of events.

When the head and body move in opposite directions, as occurs during the initial milliseconds of a collision, the body reacts quickly to try to prevent serious spinal cord injury. The strong neck muscles tighten up in a brief protective spasm triggered by the stretch reflexes, thereby supporting the spine and head and absorbing as much of the transmitted forces from the collision as possible. Whereas these "heroic" efforts by the cervical (or neck) muscles may be successful in preventing serious neurologic injuries, severe sprains of the neck muscles and ligaments may occur from the overwhelming transmitted collision forces.

Two events happen that give rise to muscle and ligament trauma and pain in a rear-end collision. First, the sudden force from behind causes forced compression and extension of the neck. This stretches and tears the front neck muscles and also causes downward pressure and compression of the structures in the back of the neck, such as ligaments and joints.

> **There is usually no correlation between the severity of the injury and how much damage was done to the car.**

Secondly, the rebound neck flexion and brief protective spasm stretch the ligaments and muscles in the back of the neck and compress the structures in the front of the neck. The stretching that occurs on the ligaments and neck muscles causes tears and injuries and results in pain. The neck, shoulders and back can suffer muscle and ligament injuries as part of the whiplash injury.

The injuries usually cause microscopic swelling or edema and hemorrhage due to disruption and tears of the muscle and ligament fibers. Usually there is no gross hemorrhage or swelling. The whiplash injury is categorized as a macroscopic trauma (see Chapter 3). Often there is no immediate pain if there is no major nerve damage. However, the microscopic damage with edema and hemorrhage causes irritation of the pain-mediating nerves and results in pain and spasms. The pain may occur in a few minutes or may not develop for a day or so, but usually some pain occurs within a few hours.

Different parts of the neck can be injured unequally depending upon the position of the head at the time of the collision or if the impact was not directly to the front or the rear but more to one side or to the other.

Additional injuries can occur if the head strikes an object such as a windshield, steering wheel or window during the collision. Secondary injuries to soft tissues can occur by sudden "slowing down" (deceleration) or "speeding up" (acceleration) forces that are superimposed on the initial whiplash injuries. Concussions or head injuries can result from serious head trauma.

> *Human tissue is extremely fragile and can be easily injured from trauma that doesn't cause damage to inorganic material such as car metal. Today's cars are better designed to absorb shock, but this shock can still damage human tissue inside the car.*

There is usually no correlation between the severity of the injury and how much damage was done to the car. Severe tissue damage and injury to the neck have been described during a collision when the offending car was moving only seven miles per hour. (Schutt and Dohan, 1968, JAMA). Human organic tissue is extremely fragile and can be easily injured from trauma that doesn't cause damage to inorganic material such as car metal. Today's cars are better designed to absorb shock, but this shock can still damage human tissue inside the car.

An example of this phenomenon is an egg inside a carton. The egg (representing biologic tissue) is protected by the egg carton (representing the car). If the egg carton were dropped to the floor, the carton would not be damaged, but upon opening it, one may find the egg to be broken. The impact from the floor still damaged the more fragile contents inside, even though the outside carton was undamaged.

Headrests don't stop neck injuries when a car is

rear-ended. A recent evaluation of head restraints in cars by the Insurance Institute for Highway Safety found that 97% of the new cars tested had headrests that could not be positioned properly or did not stay in place during a crash, thus offering little protection against neck injuries.

Various head, neck, shoulder and back injuries can result from whiplash-type trauma. The most common injury is a cervical sprain. Other common injuries include shoulder sprains, back sprains, concussions (if the head is struck), cervical disk herniation (traumatic rupture of the disk), and cervical subluxation (partial dislocation of the vertebrae). A number of people who experience whiplash injuries will ultimately develop fibromyalgia, specifically post-traumatic fibromyalgia.

> *A number of people who experience whiplash injuries will ultimately develop fibromyalgia, specifically post-traumatic fibromyalgia.*

5

The Medical History in Post-Traumatic Fibromyalgia

The medical history is an account of the events in the patient's life that have relevance to the particular problem for which the patient is seeing the doctor. In simple terms, it is what the patient tells the doctor in his or her own words. The medical history is a vital portion of the overall medical evaluation, which also includes the physical examination, review of previous medical records, and diagnostic testing, diagnosis and recommendations by the treating physician.

The medical history has various medical and legal purposes. Medical purposes include assisting the physician in making the diagnosis, enabling the physician to provide the necessary care and treatment for the patient, and to serve as a record for monitoring progress and treatment response. Legal purposes include documenting the findings for insurance claims. The medical history can serve as legal proof in cases of injury, compensation or malpractice.

The medical history is not simply an unprompted narrative by the patient, but rather a specialized form of information gathering prompted by the physician. The components of a medical history include vital statistics, chief complaint, history of present illness, past medical history, social history, family history and review of systems. Each of the components will be reviewed.

Vital statistics. This data is usually recorded by the physician's staff, such as a receptionist or medical secretary, or filled out on an information form provided the patient before seeing the doctor. Such information includes name, address, phone number, birth date, age, marital status, and occupation. Referral source (whether a patient was self-referred or referred by someone else, such as a doctor, attorney or friend) is also noted. During the actual history taking, the physician checks with the patient on the accuracy of all the prerecorded vital statistics.

> *A symptom is a subjective finding, an abnormal sensation perceived by the patient. An objective finding is a physical sign that can be seen, felt or heard by the medical examiner.*

Chief complaint. The medical history begins with a chief complaint, which is a list of one or more symptoms causing the major problem or problems for which the patient came to see the doctor. "Symptom" is a Greek word that means "anything that has befallen one." In individuals with post-traumatic fibromyalgia, the chief complaint, and hence the primary symptom, will be muscle pain. A symptom is usually considered a subjective finding, that is, an abnormal sensation perceived by the patient, as contrasted with an objective finding, which is a physical sign that can be seen, felt or heard by the medical examiner.

Complaints or symptoms are not diagnoses. The primary purpose of the chief complaint is to highlight the primary reason the patient is presenting for diagnosis and treatment recommendations, and to provide important clues for the physician in making a differential diagnosis and, ultimately, the definitive diagnosis.

History of present illness. This part is the detailed narrative of the patient's symptoms, particularly the chief complaints. This should provide a chronologic, succinct narrative that accurately describes the patient's symptoms. The history of present illness should convey a clear picture of the patient's problems and how they interfere with his or her surroundings, whether it be work, daily life activities or interpersonal relationships.

The patient's description of symptoms is clarified by precise location and time course. In addition, quantification is important to measure the severity of the symptoms by having the patient describe how they affect him or her in everyday life.

> *The history of present illness should convey a clear picture of the patient's problems and how they interfere with his or her surroundings, whether it be work, daily life activities or interpersonal relationships.*

Included in this part is a detailed account of what has happened from the beginning of the symptom to the current time, including any previous medical testing or evaluations and treatments. The physician will usually take detailed notes to place these historical events in chronological sequence and assist in making a diagnosis.

Past medical history. This section reviews the patient's health over his or her lifetime before the present illness. Often, this part does not have much significance in making the final diagnosis, although it may provide clues for the diagnosis and can be used with information from the present illness. A detailed past medical history will include information regarding previous infections, operations, injuries, hospitalizations, medications and medication allergies.

Social history. This section reviews marital history, social and economic status, education, employment and recreational activities. In addition, habits such as diet and the use of drugs, tobacco and alcohol are reviewed in the social history.

Family history. This section searches for any type of hereditary medical problem. The health of parents or siblings is briefly reviewed for medical conditions, causes of death or hereditary problems.

Review of systems. This section is primarily a search for symptoms that may have been missed during the present illness. A brief review of various organ systems, including skin, blood, eyes, lungs, heart and bowels, is performed to inquire for any symptoms that may be significant in making a final diagnosis.

> *A doctor cannot make a diagnosis based on history alone.*

Pain is the most common complaint in persons who are ultimately diagnosed with post-traumatic fibromyalgia. When taking a pain history, the doctor should ask specific questions that are important in eliciting the subjective component of pain. These questions include:

- Where is the pain?
- When did the pain start?
- What caused the pain?
- Did it start suddenly or was it a gradual occurrence with no obvious cause identified?
- Was there pain present prior to the current pain? If so, was it the same type of pain or a different pain, and was it ongoing pain or constant pain, or had the previous pain disappeared?
- Describe the pain: What does it feel like? Is it severe? Is it constant or intermittent? Does it radiate to other locations?
- What makes the pain worse? Certain positions such as sitting or standing? Bending or lifting? Other activities? Weather changes? Stress?

- What makes the pain better? Rest? Heat? Massage? Curtailing certain activities?

- How does the pain interfere with function? Does it prevent you from performing your job? Can you do work around the house? Has it caused personality changes interfering with relationships? Can you no longer do hobbies previously enjoyed?

- What testing and treatment have been done for the pain?

- Over time has the pain gotten better, worse or stayed the same?

Based on my experience in obtaining histories on hundreds of patients who were ultimately diagnosed with post-traumatic fibromyalgia, I will try to discern a "typical history" of a person with post-traumatic fibromyalgia. However, each person's history is unique and I will not devalue any patient's individual story by describing a common "generic" summary. Rather, I am alert to common themes and patterns that occur with surprising regularity in individuals who have been diagnosed with post-traumatic fibromyalgia.

There is no such thing as a diagnostic history. **A doctor cannot make a diagnosis based on history alone.** Rather, the history must be incorporated as part of the total clinical evaluation and that includes history, the exam and diagnostic testing. By reviewing charts of previous patients who have ultimately been diagnosed with fibromyalgia, I have "backtracked" so to speak, to determine what details and patterns were present in the history of these individuals that seem to be typical in post-traumatic fibromyalgia.

By backtracking and getting specific information with retrospective analysis, a medical professional can apply this information to future patients who give similar histories and make a prediction about the diagnosis. A physical examination and review of all diagnostic testing still need to occur, but the characteristic history allows the medical practitioner to include post-traumatic fibromyalgia as one of the main diagnostic considerations.

Although there is usually some history of previous pain, this was not described as pain that required ongoing treatment, nor did it cause ongoing pain and functional limitations.

What is the "typical history" in persons with post-traumatic fibromyalgia?

The person will report pain as a chief complaint. The most common areas of pain are the back of the neck, shoulders, mid-back and low-back areas. Sometimes patients say they hurt all over. The person reports that his or her pain began following a trauma, usually a motor vehicle accident. Prior to the trauma, there was no previous ongoing pain problem. There may have been an occasional headache, back strain or various aches and pains, some of which may have required medical treatment.

Although there is usually some history of previous pain, this was not described as pain that required ongoing treatment nor did it cause ongoing pain and functional limitations. The person was able to function in his or her everyday life, performing daily life skills, working full time and participating in recreational activities. Chronic pain did not limit the person's function or abilities. Previous pains were completely different from current pains, with current pains being described as more severe and persistent than those previously experienced.

What accidents would be the most common cause of injuries resulting in a post-traumatic fibromyalgia?

The rear-end collision is the most common type of motor vehicle accident. Patients describe being a belted driver who was stopped in a car that was rear-ended by another vehicle. They remember feeling their head jerk backward and then forward, and some of them may have struck their head on the rear-view mirror or window or hit the steering wheel, and they remember the seat belt locking up on them. Sometimes the head rest breaks due to the force from the rear-end collision. Loss of consciousness is not typical unless individuals hit their head hard and develop a severe head injury and concussion. There is often an initial daze or shock, and the person may have difficulty remembering exact details that happened during the first few seconds following an accident.

> *Previous pains were completely different from current pains, with current pains being described as more severe and persistent than those previously experienced.*

The individual may not notice any pain at first, but often there is a feeling of immediate discomfort: sharp pain, pressure sensation, tightness or inability to move the neck. In addition to the neck, other reported areas of pain after a rear-end collision include the back of the head, shoulders, and mid- and low-back area. Knee injuries are common as the knees often jam into the dashboard. Shoulder, elbow and wrist injuries are common as well, especially if the person locks up the arms on the steering wheel in anticipation of a rear-end collision.

Although the initial symptoms may not be considered severe, usually if there is any complaint of neck or back pain, paramedics will transport the individual to the nearest emergency room with a neck or back board in place. Some persons drive themselves or have family members take them to the hospital within a short time after the accident. Others may not go to the emergency room until later that day or even the next day when severe pain develops.

In the emergency room the person will be examined by a doctor. A history and a physical examination are performed and usually X-rays are obtained, particularly of the neck or cervical area. The X-rays do not generally show any fracture and are usually interpreted as normal. In some patients, however, there is some straightening of the normal neck curvature on the X-ray which is interpreted as loss of the normal cervical lordosis. This X-ray finding is thought to indicate neck muscle spasms or tightening causing this malpositioning or straightening of the neck.

> **Others may not go to the emergency room until later that day or even the next day when severe pain develops.**

The emergency room doctor's initial diagnosis is usually muscle sprain, i.e., cervical sprain for the neck, thoracic sprain for the mid-back, lumbar sprain for the low back, and so on.

The emergency room treatment approach includes medicines to help decrease pain, relax muscles and reduce inflammation. A cervical collar or neck brace is often prescribed. The patient will be instructed to follow up with his or her family doctor, primary care doctor or specialist if pain persists.

The day following the accident is when many people will notice their most severe pain. They often say they wake up feeling like they had been run over by a truck. They are sore everywhere including head, neck, shoulders and back. Symptoms other than pain are described, including dizziness, light-headedness, headaches and stiffness. The persistence of severe pain will cause the person to seek further medical counseling either through the primary care doctor or a specialist.

The doctor will be seen usually within a few days following the trauma. This doctor will take a history and examine the patient and usually confirm the presence of muscle sprains as a result of the accident. Additional treatments at this time may include prescription medicines, time off from work, activity restrictions, adjustments or manipulation therapy, or physical therapy.

The person who ultimately develops post-traumatic fibromyalgia will not report substantial improvement with these various treatments. Follow-up with the primary care doctor or a specialist may lead to additional testing. If headaches are a problem, a computed tomography (CAT scan) of the head may be ordered to look for abnormalities.

If neck or low-back pain is the primary source of pain, additional X-rays or magnetic resonance imaging (MRI) studies may be ordered to look at the bony structures and to look for any disk disease, such as herniation or degeneration. If pain is radiating to the arms and legs and is associated with numbness or weakness, specialized testing called electrodiagnostic testing (often referred to as an EMG) may be ordered to look for nerve damage as a result of the trauma.

Over time, the person may report some improvement of pain, but the pain never disappears. In fact, it often flares up or becomes aggravated and involves other areas of the body, even those that may not have been injured initially. Pain is described as a constant ache that varies in intensity. Numbness in the arms and legs is common. Headaches are also common, usually in the back of the neck radiating up into the head itself and perhaps turning into a migraine headache. The person will often describe sore spots that develop and that are very painful when pressed on.

With the persistence of pain in spite of various treatments, the individual may be referred to a specialist for additional evaluation and recommendation. Various specialists who treat pain disorders include physiatrists like myself, orthopedic surgeons, rheumatologists, neurologists, anesthesiologists and chiropractors.

> *Various specialists who treat pain disorders include physiatrists, orthopedic surgeons, rheumatologists, neurologists, anesthesiologists and chiropractors.*

When a "typical patient" comes to me for further evaluation and treatment, I begin the medical evaluation by obtaining a medical history. Based on a review of nearly 500 charts of patients with a diagnosis of post-traumatic fibromyalgia, I have seen far more women than men. In motor vehicle accidents, women outnumber men five to one, but in other types of traumas, the women outnumber men by only three to one. The patient ages range from 7 to 76, but most of the patients are in their 20s and 30s. Sixty percent of these patients were referred to me by another doctor, 35% were self-referred or referred by a non-physician medical professional, and 5% were referred by an attorney or friend. The average length of time from the trauma until I saw the patient for the first time ranges from one day to 15 years, with the majority not seen by me for at least three months following the trauma.

All of the patients described pain as their primary symptom. The pain is mainly in the muscles and is constant and persistent with periodic exacerbations. Other frequent symptoms include headaches, numbness, weakness, fatigue, radiating pain, stiffness and poor sleep. I take a complete history which includes a patient description of all the events and evaluations that have happened prior to seeing me.

The patients have all described trauma as the cause of their pain. Most patients are able to describe the exact moment when the trauma occurred and their pains began. (Various types of trauma are summarized in Figure 1 of Chapter 3.) I ask if any additional trauma has occurred since the original "offending" trauma, and usually the answer is no. If additional traumas have occurred, I ask if the pain changed as a result of the additional trauma, becoming more severe, affecting new locations or causing a temporary or persistent exacerbation.

As part of the description of the pain, I ask the person to tell what makes it better or worse. The person will usually describe the pain being worse when she/he does certain activities such as reaching out or overhead with the arms, trying to bend, attempting to lift objects, sitting or standing for long periods of time, and cold, damp weather. The pain may be improved temporarily with heat from a heating pad or hot shower, massage, rest, and moving around or alternating positions. Some people describe stretching and exercise as helpful, but most people describe attempts at exercise as causing increased pain.

When patients are asked to describe how the pain interferes with activities, there is usually a universal response that the pain always interferes with activities attempted since the trauma, whereas there was not a problem with these activities prior to the trauma. The person often cannot perform usual job duties without the pain interfering to some degree, particularly jobs that require a lot of reaching, bending, repetitive arm use, prolonged standing, walking, and prolonged exposure to cold, damp weather. Many people cannot perform jobs and have not been able to return to their work because of severe pain.

Recreational activities such as bowling, golfing or even a previous active exercise program such as walking or working out may be too painful to continue after the trauma. The individual simply avoids these activities altogether. Patients frequently describe inability to perform household chores such as running a sweeper, doing laundry, scrubbing floors or other activities. Interpersonal relationships may be strained due to persistent pain causing increased irritability, stress, frustration, depression and financial problems.

When asked if the pain is getting better, worse or staying the same over time, these patients consistently, as a group, divide up equally among the categories. That is, one-third of them will say their initial pain symptoms improved somewhat but continued to be severe, one-third will say that their symptoms have gotten worse over time, and one-third will say that there has been no change in their initial symptoms.

In the past medical history, it is important to determine if any previous medical conditions could potentially cause pain and be unrelated to trauma. Examples of such conditions include inflammatory arthritis, neurologic disease, diabetes, and thyroid abnormalities.

The chief complaint and history of present illness are the most important components of the medical history, although the entire medical history is obtained. In the past medical history, it is important to determine if there are any previous medical conditions that could potentially cause pain and be unrelated to trauma. Examples of such conditions include inflammatory arthritis, neurologic disease, diabetes, and thyroid abnormalities. Medications are reviewed including current and past medicines used, and it is important to note whether there are any medication allergies. Previous surgeries, particularly if they involve neck, back or disk problems or other spinal disorders are asked about.

In the social history of a patient with post-traumatic fibromyalgia, I try to determine what is the current occupational status, whether the patient is working, what job duties are required, whether restricted job duties are available and whether or not a person has been able to work. I ask if the person has lost his or her job because of the pain. I ask about use of tobacco or alcohol, and if there have been any changes consumption of these substances. Marital status, interpersonal relationships, and any lifestyle changes are reviewed here, if not discussed in the history. Also, any changes in the person's everyday activities, including daily life skills such as bathing, dressing, basic activities in the home, as well as any changes in ability to perform hobbies, recreation activities, or secondary jobs are reviewed. I try to determine what the patient wishes in terms of resuming employment or hobbies.

The family history is briefly covered. I am interested in any specific hereditary problems or conditions that can be linked to the patient's current problems, such as rheumatoid arthritis, lupus, scoliosis, and certain neurologic problems. I also ask about family history of fibromyalgia in parents, siblings, children or other family members. If no family members have been officially diagnosed with fibromyalgia, I still ask if any of these family members have symptoms and complaints similar to those of the patient.

Under the review of systems, I try to cover any areas that may not have been mentioned in the history of present illness. I ask if the bowel and bladder functions are normal, if sleep is affected, if chest pain or shortness of breath has developed. I need to know about symptoms that may be seen in fibromyalgia or may indicate additional problems that need to be considered.

A thorough medical history is an important part of the medical evaluation. Not only does it provide accurate details regarding the patient's pain symptoms, but it also enables the physician to guide his or her thinking into what possible diagnoses are to be considered and if post-traumatic fibromyalgia should be included as a major diagnostic consideration.

After the medical history is taken, the physical examination is performed.

6

The Physical Exam In Post-Traumatic Fibromyalgia

The purpose of the physical examination is to detect any abnormalities or patterns of abnormal changes that help the physician determine the diagnosis. The experienced physician recognizes both normal and abnormal findings in the physical examination and utilizes his or her knowledge of these findings to help make a diagnosis.

The clinician uses sight in inspecting the patient for any abnormalities, uses touch in palpating for any abnormalities, and uses hearing in auscultation or listening through the stethoscope for abnormalities. Devices such as a stethoscope, reflex hammer and tape measure can assist the physician in obtaining information during the physical examination. Knowledge and skills are required for the physician to recognize that various abnormal findings on the physical examination are meaningful.

In persons with pain from post-traumatic fibromyalgia, the most useful part of the physical exam is the neuromusculoskeletal examination. The nerves, muscles, and bones/joints are closely evaluated for specific normal or abnormal findings. As a physiatrist (specialist in physical medicine and rehabilitation) my training has particularly emphasized the neuromusculoskeletal examination and being able to detect abnormalities and apply meaning to them. All physicians acquire knowledge on neuromusculoskeletal examinations as part of the entire physical examination, but various specialists who treat disorders involving the nerves, muscles and bones are trained more intensively on this portion of the examination.

An abnormality detected by a physician during the physical exam is considered an objective finding. An objective finding is one that is verifiable and reproducible by the examining physician and that would be found by another physician upon examination of the same patient. Objective findings, unlike subjective complaints, do not depend on the patient's complaints. Rather, the objective finding is one determined solely by the medical examiner.

> *The person with post-traumatic fibromyalgia will have distinct and reproducible findings upon physical examination. A knowledgeable clinician will be able to detect these abnormalities, no matter how subtle they may be.*

The person with post-traumatic fibromyalgia will have distinct and reproducible findings upon physical examination. A knowledgeable clinician will be able to detect these abnormalities, no matter how subtle they may be. A person with post-traumatic fibromyalgia is not expected to have paralysis, atrophy (muscle wasting), joint swelling or redness, or loss of reflexes. However, the absence of any severe neurologic or inflammatory findings does not mean that a severe problem is not present, nor does it mean that there are no abnormal physical findings whatsoever. The physical exam findings that are present in patients with post-traumatic fibromyalgia, namely, the unique pattern of tender points, are important and diagnostic.

The main findings upon physical examination are the tender points. Tender points are areas in the soft tissues, either the muscles, tendons or ligaments, which are very sensitive and painful when pressed. These tender points are reproducible and objective findings and are in distinct locations of the body. This means that tender points do not move around, but stay in the same locations. Tender points can be found in multiple soft tissue locations of the body (muscles, tendons, ligaments).

The presence of tender points was the main criterion used to identify generalized fibromyalgia in a study by the American College of Rheumatology in 1990. According to their criteria, generalized fibromyalgia is diagnosed when an individual has a history of widespread pain and characteristic painful tender points. The pain is considered widespread when all of the following are present: pain in both sides of the body, pain above and below the waist, and pain along the spine.

In addition, there should be pain in 11 of 18 distinct tender point sites on a patient while pressing on these areas. The 18 tender points are located in 9 areas of the body, both sides. (See Figure 3.) These 18 tender points were determined to be the "signature" tender points that distinguish individuals with fibromyalgia from individuals with chronic muscle pain resulting from other causes.

FIGURE 3: TENDER POINTS DIAGRAM

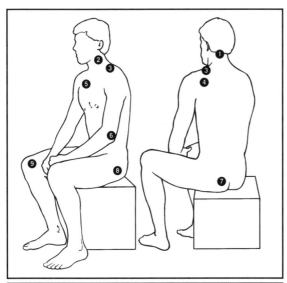

These "signature" areas include:

1. The occiput or back of the head where the neck muscles connect to the skull, known as the suboccipital muscle.

2. Low cervical muscle. This is along the neck muscle in front of the fifth, sixth and seventh cervical vertebrae.

3. Trapezius muscle. This broad muscle extends from the neck to the shoulder. The tender point is at the midpoint of the upper part of the muscle.

4. Supraspinatus muscle. This muscle is located at the top of the shoulder blade and should be painful in the part closer to the spine.

5. The second rib. This costochondral area is right below the collar bone.

6. Lateral epicondyle. This is located at the top of the forearm and is also called the tennis-elbow area.

7. Outer gluteus maximus. This is the buttock muscle and should be painful in the upper outer portion.

8. Greater trochanter. This is part of the femur or thigh bone which has a knobby protrusion right below the hip joint, covered by a bursa (fluid-filled sac).

9. Medial knee. This painful area is right above the inside of the knee.

These nine areas on each side of the body (total of 18 tender points) were found to be the key locations to palpate in generalized fibromyalgia.

> *The absence of any severe neurologic or inflammatory findings does not mean that a severe problem is not present, nor does it mean that there are no abnormal physical findings whatsoever.*

Palpation is the art of using the sense of touch to feel for abnormalities. The tips of the fingers and thumbs are the medical examiner's most sensitive "instruments" for examining the soft tissues for the presence of painful tender points. I prefer to use my thumbs while palpating.

A positive tender point is one that, upon palpation with enough pressure to cause my thumbnail to blanch (about 4 kilograms of force), and causes a consistent painful response in the patient. The patient may withdraw and try to avoid the pressure, or may indicate that the palpation hurts in that location. The physician examines all body soft tissue areas.

> *Muscles that have developed fibromyalgia have a peculiar consistency that feels like nylon bands or little nodules when they are rubbed deeply.*

Tender points can be found essentially in any muscle but usually occur in larger muscles including neck, shoulder, mid-back, low-back and hip muscles. Particular emphasis is placed on palpating the characteristic or signature tender point areas described above, but the tender points in fibromyalgia are not limited to these areas. The presence of tender points is confirmed by both reproducing the painful patient reaction with the appropriate pressure upon palpation and by determining abnormal muscle consistency that is usually present in the tender points.

What exactly do these tender points feel like? The muscles that have developed fibromyalgia have a peculiar consistency that feels like nylon bands or little nodules when they are rubbed deeply. This band-like or ropy consistency is an important abnormal finding in persons with post-traumatic fibromyalgia. Sometimes these taut bands or ropiness involve a larger area and form a fibromyalgia nodule or firm lump that can be palpated in the muscle. The tender points have this type of nodular or firm-lump consistency that feels like tight hard muscle instead of the normal firm gel-like consistency of normal muscle.

This tightness, ropiness or nodular consistency that can be detected with palpation represents localized muscle spasms. When groups of muscle fibers go into spasms, an experienced physician will be able to palpate this firm bundle and appreciate this as a localized muscle spasm. If these localized spasms form consistent painful taut bands or nodules, a tender point may be present. These nodules can vary in size depending on whether the muscle is having more or less localized spasms, but it is my experience that these tender points or nodules never completely disappear once fibromyalgia has developed. Further discussion of the cause of post-traumatic fibromyalgia occurs in Chapter 9.

> *Seemingly unrelated body parts are linked together neurologically because they arose from a common tissue during the body's embryonic stage. Thus, these common tissues always "share" a neurologic link by small sensory nerve fibers and can "communicate" with each other in certain situations.*

If pressing on a tender area causes pain, numbness or tingling that radiates or spreads to a different area, this painful spot is called a trigger point. A trigger point is another typical finding in patients with post-traumatic fibromyalgia. As an example, if a medical examiner pressed on a tender area in the trapezius, and the patient felt numbness radiating down the entire arm into the hand, that area in the trapezius muscle would be called a trigger point. Trigger points are also common in myofascial pain syndrome (see Chapter 1), which I believe is a condition synonymous with regional fibromyalgia.

These trigger points can cause confusion since they mimic a pinched nerve. However, the nerve is not being pinched. Rather the trigger areas in the muscles cause radiating symptoms to distant locations.

Seemingly unrelated body parts are linked together neurologically because they arose from a common tissue during the body's embryonic stage. Thus, these common tissues always "share" a neurologic link by small sensory nerve fibers and can "communicate" with each other in certain situations. For example, when an individual is having a heart attack, he may experience numbness in the left arm. There is no problem with the left arm, per se; rather, the heart muscle is being damaged, but because it has embryonic connections with the left arm, it sends referred symptoms down the left arm. The injured heart muscle acts as a trigger point in this situation.

> *If pressing on a tender area causes pain, numbness or tingling that radiates or spreads to a different area, this painful spot is called a trigger point.*

There are hundreds of potential trigger points in the body. Individuals with post-traumatic fibromyalgia can develop trigger points because the painful areas in the muscles, i.e., tender points, can activate the muscles' small sensory nerves and refer their signals to distant yet neurologically related territories. Trigger points can occur after an injury and cause a person to feel numbness, pain or altered sensations.

In the head and neck area, there are many potential trigger points that can cause referred headaches, light-headedness, dizziness, jaw pain and ringing in the ears. In the neck and back many trigger points can refer symptoms to the arms or legs. These trigger points may be irritated or activated after a trauma.

Pressing on these trigger points during the exam will cause enough irritation to "activate" them. If the medical examiner can reproduce the patient's subjective arm numbness by palpating a trigger point, this provides valuable information as to the exact cause of the numbness.

Another frequent physical finding in post-traumatic fibromyalgia is dermatographism, also known as "skin writing." Scratching with the finger along the skin will cause a red mark or rash to form in patients with dermatographism. This phenomenon is most pronounced in the skin overlying painful muscles in individuals with post-traumatic fibromyalgia.

> *Another frequent physical finding in post-traumatic fibromyalgia is dermatographism, also known as "skin writing." Scratching with the finger along the skin will cause a red mark or rash to form in patients with dermatographism.*

Dermatographism occurs because the skin is hypersensitive due to the small autonomic nerves becoming dysfunctional or hyperactive in post-traumatic fibromyalgia. The autonomic nerves are the small nerves that mediate sensation such as pain, tingling, numbness and temperature to the skin and other organs. They control blood flow to the skin, among other functions.

Another physical exam abnormality which is caused by autonomic nervous system dysfunction is the presence of decreased sensation. During sensory testing in the physical examination using light-touch sensation, pinprick sensation or even a vibration sensation, the patient with post-traumatic fibromyalgia may notice decreased sensation in certain areas of the body, usually in the arms or legs. One side may be more affected than the other depending on the trauma.

For example, an individual with a lot of right neck and shoulder pain may complain of numbness in the right arm, and upon sensory testing, there is decreased light touch and pinprick sensation on the right arm compared to the left. The person will still be able to feel light touch or sharp sensations on the affected arm. The decreased sensation tends to affect the entire arm, not a specific territory of the arm, as would be expected if a nerve root or larger peripheral nerve were affected. The smaller autonomic nerve signals to this area are dysfunctional and cause these detectable sensory abnormalities on the physical exam.

Still another finding that I note frequently in patients with post-traumatic fibromyalgia, and that I believe is part of the autonomic nervous system dysfunction, is the presence of "goosebumps" upon examination of patients with post-traumatic fibromyalgia. These are usually noticed in the legs during the palpation exam after various painful tender points have been pressed. These goosebumps, technically known as piloerections, result when the autonomic nervous system signals the hair to stand up on the skin. This finding is not present in everyone with fibromyalgia, but I rarely see it in an individual who does not have fibromyalgia.

Another common physical exam abnormality is decreased joint range of motion due to painful, tense muscles. Full joint flexibility depends on the muscle's ability to relax and allow the joint to achieve full motion. If the muscles are not able to relax because of tightness and localized spasms, as occurs with fibromyalgia, the joints may not be able to achieve their full range. This limitation of joint motion can be detected and objectively reproduced on physical examination. The neck, shoulders and low back are the most common joints with decreased range of motion in post-traumatic fibromyalgia.

Of all the exam findings indicated above, the painful tender points are the most important and meaningful physical finding in the diagnosis of post-traumatic fibromyalgia. Without these positive tender points, the diagnosis of post-traumatic fibromyalgia can not be made.

The presence of the other abnormal physical exam findings is important but not as meaningful as the tender points. The tender points and associated localized muscle spasms, when combined with the trigger points, dermatographism, decreased sensation, piloerections and decreased range of motion, are all considered valuable objective findings. They strongly suggest post-traumatic fibromyalgia, particularly if there is an appropriate history.

> **If abnormal physical findings such as neurologic abnormalities or joint inflammation are present, then something other than post-traumatic fibromyalgia is present in the patient.**

The physical examination of a person who is ultimately diagnosed with post-traumatic fibromyalgia will not reveal the following abnormalities:

- True neurologic weakness
- Abnormal loss of reflexes
- Joint swelling, heat or inflammation
- Abnormal thyroid swelling or associated clinical thyroid abnormalities
- Abnormal muscle neurologic tone called spasticity
- Atrophy or wasting of muscles

Other than the tender points, localized muscle spasms, trigger points, autonomic nerve findings and decreased range of motion, the rest of the physical exam in post-traumatic fibromyalgia is within normal limits. If abnormal physical findings such as neurologic abnormalities or joint inflammation are present, then something other than post-traumatic fibromyalgia is present in the patient.

Because fibromyalgia does not cause obvious physical exam abnormalities with inspection and the patient looks "normal," it has often been termed "The Invisible Condition." As we have determined, however, an experienced physician examiner will be able to detect the subtle yet definite abnormalities upon physical examination, even when there are no obvious abnormalities upon inspection. The diagnosis of post-traumatic fibromyalgia is made when the medical examiner incorporates the history and exam findings and any diagnostic testing to explain the patient's clinical picture.

> *Because fibromyalgia does not cause obvious physical exam abnormalities with inspection and the patient looks "normal," it has often been termed "The Invisible Condition."*

How soon after an injury do these typical tender points and other physical findings develop? Most soft-tissue injuries, if they were to completely heal, do so within six weeks. Some severe soft-tissue injuries can take up to four months or longer to heal, but if a soft-tissue injury has not healed within six months, then the probability is very high that the condition has become a chronic and permanent one.

Using this information, I do not think a definitive diagnosis of post-traumatic fibromyalgia should be made until at least six months after the injury. This time frame "rule of thumb" will allow adequate time for full spontaneous healing to occur. This is not to say that the painful tender points are not present earlier than six months. Indeed I have detected them within a month of the trauma. But the tender points usually take time to fully evolve and if they are still present six months following the trauma, then I can state within a reasonable degree of medical certainty that they are chronic and permanent. If the total picture is consistent with post-traumatic fibromyalgia, then it can be stated that post-traumatic has become chronic and permanent as well.

The longer one's pain persists following a trauma and the longer the tender points are present after the trauma, the higher the probability that this person's condition will evolve into the more chronic and permanent post-traumatic fibromyalgia. Once the condition has established itself (it can take anywhere from a few months to six months but shouldn't be diagnosed until at least six months as I have indicated above), it is a permanent condition.

> *I do not think a definitive diagnosis of post-traumatic fibromyalgia should be made until at least six months after the injury. This is not to say that the painful tender points are not present earlier than six months.*

Even if a medical examiner first sees a patient months or even years later, the characteristic painful tender points should continue to be present and enable a diagnosis of post-traumatic fibromyalgia to be made within a reasonable degree of medical certainly.

The physical exam abnormalities in patients with post-traumatic fibromyalgia are considered objective findings, that is, they are discreet, verifiable and reproducible abnormal physical findings. Individuals without fibromyalgia will not have pain or tender points during palpation of the designated anatomical areas.

When I examine patients, I verify the reproducibility of tender points by repeated palpation of these anatomic areas during the physical exam. A painful tender point will always elicit the same patient response and have the same abnormal muscle consistency whenever palpated. I also verify the tender points by distracting the person away from my palpating fingers. For example, I may divert the patient's attention to my other hand while applying consistent pressure with the palpating hand over the suspected painful tender point. Patients with reproducible objective tender points will readily indicate pain in the tender point area even with distraction attempts. With these techniques, the probability is low that any individual can pretend to have fibromyalgia, no matter how knowledgeable he or she may be about this condition.

> *The probability is low that any individual can pretend to have fibromyalgia, no matter how knowledgeable he or she may be about this condition.*

Fibromyalgia has been termed "The Invisible Condition" because the person appears normal; he or she has no obvious abnormalities. However, an experienced examiner will be able to detect the signature objective findings and discover the cause of the hidden pain.

7

Diagnostic Testing in Post-Traumatic Fibromyalgia

There is no single testing procedure that is diagnostic of post-traumatic fibromyalgia. In fact, routine labs and other tests are normal in fibromyalgia. There are specialized tests on which fibromyalgia patients test positive, but these tests are not considered routine and are often done only in specialized labs or centers.

A normal lab or test result does not mean that a specific condition such as fibromyalgia does not exist; rather, a normal result simply means that that particular test did not detect any abnormalities. Along the same line of thinking, an abnormal test does not indicate that a particular condition is present unless the medical doctor correlates the abnormality with the clinical history and physical examination.

Any diagnostic test in medicine has its limitations. Each test measures a particular unit. It may tell whether this unit is present or not, or what quantity it is present in, or how it is functioning, or what it looks like. Depending on what test is being done and what is being measured, the physician may be able to make certain diagnoses or rule them out, but each test is limited by what it is capable of measuring.

Another testing limitation is that not everyone with a particular disease will test "abnormal" for it, and some normal people (without the disease) will test "positive" for it. When an individual has a disease but tests normal, we call this test a false negative (it should have tested positive). When a test is positive, but the person really doesn't have the disease, we call this test a false positive (it should have tested negative).

> **There is no single testing procedure that is diagnostic of post-traumatic fibromyalgia.**

In medicine, we recognize that there is no test that is 100% accurate in its ability to detect an abnormality (sensitivity) or in its ability to find an abnormality with a particular condition (specificity). We have many tests that are very sensitive and specific, approaching the upper 90% in accuracy, and other tests that are a not as sensitive or specific, with no better than 50% accuracy. It is important to remember these testing limitations in interpreting all of the available information (history, exam and lab testing) and in making a final diagnosis.

An individual with post-traumatic fibromyalgia will often have various medical diagnostic tests performed after the trauma. Various categories of diagnostic testing include X-rays, special radiographic imaging, laboratory studies and electrical studies. Each test measures something different. Below is a brief review of these common categories of testing.

X-rays

X-rays are perhaps the most common diagnostic tests ordered after an acute trauma. X-rays are pictures that tell us whether the bones have normal density, whether there is a fracture, whether the bones are in proper position, or whether a foreign object (such as metal or glass) is present.

In a person who ultimately has post-traumatic

fibromyalgia, initial X-rays following a motor vehicle accident trauma, for example, may include the neck or cervical spine, the mid-back or thoracic spine, the low back or lumbar sacral spine. If the head was struck, there may be skull X-rays obtained as well. In injuries that cause post-traumatic fibromyalgia, routine or plain X-rays will be normal in the majority of cases. Even in acute injuries such as sprains or strains, there will be no evidence of fractures or abnormal bone density. If a fracture is present, then the individual has more than just a sprain; there is also a fracture.

> *A normal lab or test does not mean a specific condition such as fibromyalgia does not exist; rather, a normal result simply means that that particular test did not detect any abnormalities.*

X-rays are not diagnostic of sprains. There may be some abnormal positioning of the bones on X-rays which give clues that something has occurred in the soft tissues, such as the muscles, ligaments or disks (enclosed gelatinous substance between the vertebrae).

Often, cervical spine X-rays taken shortly after an accident reveal abnormal straightening of the bones. A normal cervical spine has a curvature to it called a lordosis. If a muscle sprain has occurred and muscle spasms have resulted, there may be straightening of the cervical spine which will show up on the cervical X-ray as a straightening or a reversal of the normal cervical lordosis. This abnormal finding is suggestive of cervical muscle spasm, but the muscles cannot be seen on the X-rays; thus the X-rays themselves are not diagnostic of any muscle spasms.

Sometimes the space between the vertebrae is narrowed on spine X-rays. This may provide a clue that a traumatic rupture of the disk between the vertebrae has occurred, causing the gelatinous substance to leak out and resulting in loss of space between the two vertebrae. Again, the spine X-ray does not show a ruptured disk; rather, it shows two vertebrae being closer to each other than normal and provides a clue that perhaps something else is going on. Individuals with post-traumatic fibromyalgia can also have a ruptured disk as a result of the trauma, but this rarely happens.

> *In post-traumatic fibromyalgia, CAT scans and MRI images are almost always normal. If they are abnormal, something other than post-traumatic fibromyalgia or something in addition to post-traumatic fibromyalgia is present.*

Special Radiographic Imaging

Computed tomography (CAT scan). A CAT scanner uses thousands of small X-ray beams to take picture "slices" of the part being tested. A computer then generates an image that combines all these "slices" of pictures to form a whole picture of the body part. This picture can show brain white and gray matter, blood, ruptured disks, fractured bones and more. A CAT scan can be taken of the head to look for a brain hemorrhage, for example, after a concussion. The cervical, thoracic and lumbar spine could also be evaluated by CAT scan to look for a herniated or ruptured disk, ligament tear or swelling.

In post-traumatic fibromyalgia, the CAT scans are almost always normal. If they are abnormal, something other than post-traumatic fibromyalgia or something in addition to post-traumatic fibromyalgia is present.

Magnetic resonance imaging (MRI). This specialized imaging is accomplished by placing the patient in a powerful magnetic field, then beaming radio waves into the field which cause tissue particles to orient themselves in a specific pattern in the magnetic field. The images generated by the

MRI machines are remarkably sharp and defined and give detailed pictures of the anatomy of the spine, soft tissues and organs, depending on what part is being scanned. This testing has become a valuable tool in the diagnosis of various disorders, but in post-traumatic fibromyalgia, the MRI is usually completely normal. The MRI, like the CAT scan, looks at the anatomy and whether there are any abnormal or damaged body parts.

Bone Scan. This specialized imaging study uses labeled calcium particles injected into the patient's blood stream. These tagged particles are taken up by the bone. If the bone is inflamed in a particular area or if it is growing more rapidly than surrounding bone, more labeled calcium particles will accumulate there. These abnormal "hot spots" can be visualized with the bone scanning.

Individuals with post-traumatic fibromyalgia will have negative bone scans; that is, no "hot spots" will be identified.

Myelogram. A myelogram is performed when a dye is injected into the spinal column in the low back. The dye fills up the spinal fluid spaces that surround the spinal cord and nerve roots. When an X-ray picture is taken, this dye shows up on the film and gives an anatomical view of the spinal cord and nerve root areas. Any abnormality within the spaces, particularly if there is any protruding or herniated disks pressing on certain nerves, can be detected.

Myelograms are normal in patients with post-traumatic fibromyalgia. If a person has an abnormal myelogram, then something other than post-traumatic fibromyalgia needs to be diagnosed. The additional diagnosis, whether it be herniated disk or spinal stenosis, will depend on the specific abnormality detected on the myelogram.

Laboratory Studies

Laboratory studies are often done on patients with persistent pain to look for any abnormalities in the body's electrolytes, muscle enzymes, bone enzymes or other areas that might provide clues as to the source of the pain. For example, persons who have chronic pain from rheumatoid arthritis will usually demonstrate abnormal laboratory studies that measure rheumatoid arthritis. The patient's hemoglobin and hematocrit (red blood count) might be low, the sedimentation rate high, and the rheumatoid factor will often be high. There are hundreds of lab tests that measure the body's major functions, but the physician will select which ones would give the most useful information for a given patient's particular problem.

> *Hundreds of lab tests can measure the body's major functions, but the physician will select which ones would give the most useful information for a given patient's particular problem.*

Routine lab tests would include a complete blood count, electrolytes, liver labs, kidney labs and body proteins. These routine labs would screen major body functions for possible diseases.

If a rheumatologic disease is suspected, more specialized labs can be ordered. Additional labs might include a sedimentation rate, a lupus lab (an antinuclear antibody or ANA), rheumatoid factor or a complement analysis. If a hormonal problem is suspected, thyroid studies, cortisol or glucose labs could be measured. The purpose of this section is not to review in detail each of the tests mentioned, but rather to introduce how tests are ordered to look for specific abnormalities or conditions. There is no routine lab test to measure fibromyalgia or post-traumatic fibromyalgia.

Electrical Studies

X-ray studies measure anatomy and lab tests measure the presence and quantity of a body unit. Electrical studies are different in that they measure the function of certain body organs. Persons with chronic or persistent pain may undergo various electrical studies to look for any measurable functional abnormalities.

Electroencephalogram (EEG). This test is used to evaluate the brainwave changes caused by certain diseases and to study sleep patterns. Various electrodes are attached to the scalp, and a machine measures the electrical currents and activities of the brain's nerves. Individuals with headaches or concussions may show some abnormalities, but individuals who have headaches as part of post-traumatic fibromyalgia will have a normal EEG.

A particular EEG test, the sleep study, measures brain activity during various sleep cycles. In fibromyalgia, including post-traumatic fibromyalgia, the majority of individuals demonstrate a characteristic sleep abnormality where the deep part of sleep, stage 4 sleep, is abnormal. This abnormality can be detected with a sleep study EEG test and supports the diagnosis of fibromyalgia, although conditions other than fibromyalgia can cause this particular type of sleep abnormality.

Electrodiagnosis. This specialized test measures the function of nerves and muscles. There are several categories of electrodiagnosis. Nerve conduction studies use small electrical shocks to stimulate nerves and record their function by measuring the time it takes for a signal to travel down the nerve, and the size of the nerve's response. Electromyography (EMG) uses a needle electrode to examine muscle and determine if there is abnormal muscle, or if the nerves to the muscles are not working normally. Evoked potentials studies use small electric shocks to measure the long pathways of nerves from a limb to the brain.

Electrodiagnostic testing measures nerve and muscle function. This type of testing can detect damaged nerves that occur when a herniated or ruptured disk pinches a nerve and causes a radiculopathy. It can detect damage to the small nerves that occur in a peripheral neuropathy. Abnormalities in the spinal cord conduction can be detected to look for certain neurologic conditions such as multiple sclerosis. Various disorders of muscles such as a myopathy or myositis can be detected with this testing.

> *Electrodiagnostic testing measures nerve and muscle function. It can detect nerve damage from a herniated disk or peripheral neuropathy, certain neurologic conditions such as multiple sclerosis or various disorders of muscles.*

Electrodiagnosis is not abnormal in all conditions that cause pain. In fact, individuals with fibromyalgia and post-traumatic fibromyalgia demonstrate normal routine electrodiagnostic testing. Fibromyalgia does not cause pinched nerves or muscle inflammation or damage of pressure on the larger nerves; therefore one would expect the electrodiagnostic testing to be normal in these individuals. Sleep studies, as mentioned earlier, can be abnormal in post-traumatic fibromyalgia.

Some investigators have studied the tender and trigger points in post-traumatic fibromyalgia using special electrical techniques and have reported an abnormal electrical pattern in the tender and trigger points. However, these reported abnormalities have not been universally found by other investigators. For that reason it is uncertain whether there are actual measurable electrical abnormalities in these fibromyalgia areas measurable using specialized techniques. It is widely accepted, however, that routine electrodiagnostic studies will be normal in individuals with fibromyalgia.

Electrocardiogram (EKG). This test measures the electrical function of the cardiac muscle (the heart) and may be ordered in individuals with chest pain. In individuals with post-traumatic fibromyalgia who have chest pain, the EKGs are normal because the chest pain is not due to cardiac muscle or heart involvement; rather, the chest muscles and soft tissues around the ribs are causing the pain.

> *Other abnormal tests also occur in fibromyalgia, but not in 100% of the patients.*

These routine categories of diagnostic testing are usually normal in individuals with post-traumatic fibromyalgia. As I have mentioned, people with post-traumatic fibromyalgia can also have other conditions and routine testing can demonstrate abnormalities that ultimately lead to this additional diagnosis. None of those tests mentioned is specific for post-traumatic fibromyalgia.

Abnormal Tests in Post-Traumatic Fibromyalgia

Even though these tests are usually normal, and no "diagnostic" test exists for fibromyalgia, there have been numerous diagnostic testing abnormalities described in fibromyalgia. Abnormal sleep studies and possibly electrical abnormalities in the tender points have been mentioned. Other abnormal tests also occur in fibromyalgia, but not in 100% of the patients. These tests are usually very specialized and done only in a few places in the country under research conditions, and thus are not considered standard, routine tests. Following is a brief summary of some of the abnormal tests in fibromyalgia.

Substance P. This is a small protein neurotransmitter that is found in the spinal column. It has several purposes, including transmission of pain signals, and may even have a protective mechanism in trying to block the continuous feedback of pain signals. In people with fibromyalgia, substance P has been found in extremely high concentrations, well above normal values.

Serotonin. Serotonin is a neurotransmitter and hormone in the brain which is usually low in patients with fibromyalgia. Serotonin is important in the brain's ability to control pain, maintain an upbeat mood or outlook, be motivated, and attend to and concentrate on a task. Serotonin has been described as the "brightness switch" of the brain, and a low serotonin level is equivalent to turning the "brightness switch" down.

Low serotonin is also closely related to clinical depression, so it is not surprising that up to half of the people with fibromyalgia will have clinical depression over the course of their fibromyalgia.

Growth hormone and growth hormone release factor (GHRF). The pituitary gland secretes growth hormone, one of the "master" hormones in the body. It directs a lot of functions, including breakdown of fat tissue and build-up of proteins. Both growth hormone and GHRF are low in fibromyalgia. GHRF is manufactured by the hypothalamus, a part of the brain that is closely linked to the hormonal system in the body and stimulates the pituitary gland to release growth hormone.

Neuropeptide Y. This small protein is a breakdown of the hormone norepinephrine, which is another brain hormone. Neuropeptide Y has been found to be low in people with fibromyalgia, indicating that norepinephrine is also low. Norepinephrine is like the "contrast switch" of the brain, helping the brain focus and give undivided attention to a particular task.

Tilt table test. This test has been found to be abnormal in some people with fibromyalgia. The individual lies down flat on a table and blood pressure and pulse are measured. The table is then slowly tilted up, and blood pressure and pulse are measured again. In people with fibromyalgia, a low pulse pressure has been found, which is the difference between the systolic and diastolic blood pressure.

> *With ongoing research, refinement and commercialization of some of these tests, we may someday see a specific test that is accepted as a good marker for fibromyalgia.*

This is thought to represent reduced sympathetic nervous system activity in people with fibromyalgia, causing inability to respond to stress. In the case of the tilt table test, the stress is gravity acting upon the nervous system.

Various other tests have been shown to be abnormal in many people with fibromyalgia. Studies have shown a lower concentration of energy-rich proteins and a lower concentration of oxygen in muscles in fibromyalgia. Magnesium, a key mineral in the biochemical process of converting oxygen in the muscle to energy, has been found to be low in muscles of persons with fibromyalgia.

As mentioned above, none of these tests is 100% specific for fibromyalgia; that is, not everyone who has abnormalities in these tests will have fibromyalgia. In addition, none of the tests is 100% sensitive for fibromyalgia; that is, someone with fibromyalgia can test normally with these specialized tests. With ongoing research, refinement and commercialization of some of these tests, we may soon see a specific test that is accepted as a good marker for fibromyalgia. Such a test does not exist at this time.

8

Diagnosing Post-Traumatic Fibromyalgia

The diagnosis of post-traumatic fibromyalgia is never assumed before a patient is seen or from the patient's history. When I see patients for the first time, I perform an independent and complete history and physical examination regardless of whether they have been previously diagnosed with post-traumatic fibromyalgia or another condition. I make no assumptions when I first see a patient. In fact, when a person with pain sees me, I always want to make sure that a potentially deadly cause of pain such as cancer is not missed. Any medical examiner needs to consider all possible causes of pain when seeing a patient and not automatically assume that any particular condition is present.

In order for a physician to diagnose post-traumatic fibromyalgia, information from the overall clinical picture (including a history, a physical exam, review of previous records, and any diagnostic testing) needs to be analyzed. The doctor can then make a diagnosis based on the total clinical picture. The final diagnosis is like a puzzle that is formed from different pieces put together to reveal the "big picture." Post-traumatic fibromyalgia requires specific pieces of the puzzle that have to fit together to form a unique "big picture."

The key features in the patient's history with post-traumatic fibromyalgia are included in the following table:

TABLE 2: SUMMARY OF KEY FEATURES OF PATIENT HISTORY

No pain complaints	prior to the trauma similar to those experienced since the trauma
A history of a trauma	whether it be an acute sudden trauma (macroscopic) or a cumulative, repetitive-type trauma (microscopic)
Pain resulting from the trauma that has persisted ever since the trauma	The pain may have improved, stayed the same or even worsened, or it may have improved temporarily and flared up. It may have had multiple treatments, but the pain has never disappeared completely and continues to be a reported problem.
Pain persisting for at least six months following a trauma	Even though the initial trauma ultimately causes fibromyalgia, one must wait at least six months from the onset of the trauma to definitely diagnose post-traumatic fibromyalgia. This span of time allows those with pain who will not develop post-traumatic fibromyalgia to heal and have their pain disappear. Healing will usually occur within six weeks, but can take up to several months. By six months the major healing of soft tissues, sprains or other injuries would have occurred.

Key features of the physical examination include:

TABLE 3: SUMMARY OF KEY EXAM FEATURES

The presence of characteristic painful tender points.	Individuals with post-traumatic fibromyalgia will often have at least 11 of 18 painful tender points according to the previously described criteria, especially if the condition has been present for over a year. However, many will have tender points that are localized only to the region of their injuries rather than in a generalized distribution. Therefore, if tender points are consistent, reproducible and in a pattern where the injuries occur, then the individual with fewer than 11 of 18 tender points will have regional fibromyalgia.
The presence of palpable localized muscle spasms (ropy muscles, nodules)	The majority of painful tender points will demonstrate palpable localized muscle spasms.
The absence of any physical exam findings that indicate a significant neuro-logic disease or rheumatologic inflammation	Examples of these exam findings would include loss of reflexes, true muscle weakness, joint swelling or heat, and muscle atrophy.
Reproducible findings upon subsequent examinations	Redemonstrating the initial tender points upon follow-up examination is a reliable and supportive physical finding of post-traumatic fibromyalgia. Also, demon-strating that more tender points are present on the fol-low-up examination than at the initial examination is supportive of the fact that regional post-traumatic fibromyalgia is becoming more generalized.

Review of the previous medical records before the patient sees a particular specialist can be helpful in making the diagnosis of post-traumatic fibromyalgia. These previous records will provide documentations of history, exams and medical diagnostic tests that were done prior to a particular follow-up specialist examination. The previous records will support and complement the patient's history and provide documentation of an "unbroken" chain of events surrounding the patient's pain complaints that began following the trauma and continued to the present time of the specialist's examination.

Previous physician records may even indicate that post-traumatic fibromyalgia has been diagnosed already, which would be consistent with the specialist's conclusion, especially if he or she also diagnosed post-traumatic fibromyalgia. Results of previously performed tests can be reviewed so that normal results can be confirmed and to avoid repeating the tests.

Diagnostic tests are not necessary to make a diagnosis of post-traumatic fibromyalgia. However, reviewing previous diagnostic testing results or obtaining additional diagnostic tests can rule out other possible conditions that cause pain and confirm that the results were all "normal." These normal results are what would be expected in post-traumatic fibromyalgia.

Before making a diagnosis of post-traumatic fibromyalgia, the doctor will carefully consider all of these key pieces of the puzzle. No assumptions are made. Instead, everything needs to be supported by the key pieces of information. Because the clinical findings of post-traumatic fibromyalgia persist for many months and years after an initial trauma, a reliable clinical examination can occur even if the doctor does not see the person for the first time for many months following the trauma. Thus the

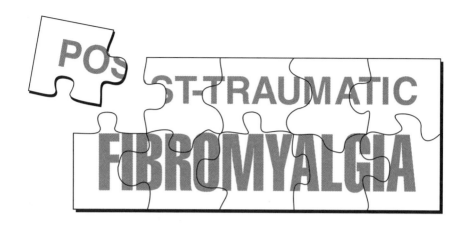

ability to diagnose post-traumatic fibromyalgia is
not dependent upon the person being seen immediately after the trauma. If the pieces of the puzzle
fit and form the unique "big picture," the diagnosis
of post-traumatic fibromyalgia can be made by the
physician.

9

Mechanisms of Post-Traumatic Fibromyalgia

As the name indicates, trauma is the cause of post-traumatic fibromyalgia. Controlled scientific studies "proving" that trauma causes fibromyalgia have not been done yet. This "burden of scientific proof" standard is frequently not met in medical conditions, even though we are able to show definite clinical relationships. For example, physicians knew clinically that cigarette smoking caused lung cancer long before scientific studies "proved" it. Another example is a drug that causes a side effect by an unknown mechanism; there is a clinical relationship between the drug and the side effect, but no scientific proof.

Likewise, there is a clinical relationship between trauma and fibromyalgia. We do not know the exact pathophysiologic mechanism or sequence of abnormal events that occur at the cellular level and ultimately lead to fibromyalgia. However, we do know that trauma can lead to fibromyalgia. In medicine, we seek exact answers and explanations, but many conditions we treat do not have "100% exact" known mechanisms.

In law, one has to show that something caused a condition with reasonable probability or within a reasonable degree of medical certainty. This does not mean 100% absolute certainty, but rather something 51% or more certain. Thus, if the trauma caused a condition like post-traumatic fibromyalgia to develop and require treatments, and if it's very unlikely that the person ever would have developed pain or needed treatments if the trauma had never happened, then legal causation (reasonable probability and medical certainty) is met.

> **If the trauma caused a condition like post-traumatic fibromyalgia to develop and require treatments, and if it's very unlikely that the person ever would have developed pain or needed treatments if the trauma had never happened, then legal causation (reasonable probability and medical certainty) is met.**

Even if we don't know the exact mechanisms of fibromyalgia, we know a lot about the condition. Various abnormalities have been found. It is difficult to look at a single abnormality and try to predict its role in the overall fibromyalgia picture. That single abnormality may interplay with multiple cells and chemicals in the body, where other abnormalities may be present also. Trying to sort out what happens first or what plays the most important role is like the proverbial "What came first, the chicken or the egg?" Measured abnormalities have to be looked at from two perspectives; are they the cause, or are they the consequences of fibromyalgia?

Before one attempts to understand the mechanism of post-traumatic fibromyalgia, it is helpful to understand normal body functions involving the muscles and their interactions with other cells of the body.

1. In a "normal" person (who does not have fibromyalgia), blood flows through the capillaries or microcirculation into the body's cells, bringing adequate supplies of oxygen, glucose and other nutrients.

2. Each cell has an electrical pump that creates a normal electrical field in the cells by moving particles with electrical charges in and out of the cells at a proper ratio.

3. Adequate amounts of the body's primary energy molecule called ATP are manufactured to fuel all the body's physiologic functions.

4. Normal amounts of hormones and neurotransmitters are present and perform their proper function.

5. The body's neurologic systems, particularly the small autonomic or sympathetic nerves, are properly coordinating nerve signals, hormone releases and capillary blood flow without overreacting.

The manufacture of proteins and hormones occurs in an orderly fashion as the body utilizes its stored glucose and fat cells. Muscles at their normal baseline are relaxed and when they are called into action, they contract efficiently and then return to a relaxed state.

This "normal" baseline is genetically determined and is expected in the human body. Not everyone inherits the same normal building blocks or genetic makeup and will have variations in the composition of the cell, particularly the protein component. Even though an individual may have normally functioning cells, there are still variations among individuals where some cells are in the low normal range and others are in the high normal range. The variation causes some body functions to just barely be done normally, whereas others are done normally with a lot of leeway or reserve function.

Many diseases are the result of inherited defects or altered genetic makeup, and fibromyalgia may be a syndrome that is largely determined by genetic predisposition.

Various studies have supported that fibromyalgia may have an inherited component. Certain protein deviations can be present at birth through these inherited genes and lead to eventual fibromyalgia. Fibromyalgia can take years to fully develop and may depend on various factors, including the presence of trauma. Other individuals with the genetic predisposition may never develop a clinical picture of fibromyalgia even though the tendency or risk is there.

> *Variations occur among normally functioning individuals, where some individuals' cells are in the low normal range and others are in the high normal range. The variation causes some body functions to just barely be done normally, whereas others are done normally with a lot of reserve function.*

In others with the genetic predisposition, an event may occur that causes fibromyalgia. Such events could include an infection (either viral or bacterial), surgery, insect bite or trauma. "Something happens" during this event that causes permanent changes in the body's function at the cellular level, and the end result of this permanent change is fibromyalgia. If trauma is involved, it is called post-traumatic fibromyalgia.

Various theories hypothesize certain events that may occur in the development of fibromyalgia following a trauma. In response to the trauma, the soft tissues undergo changes, and the previous pain-free balance in the body is permanently disrupted; post-traumatic fibromyalgia is the outcome. What may be happening in response to the actual trauma?

The soft tissues of the body, including the muscles, respond to trauma by a process called inflammation. At the site of injury in the muscles, there is disruption of cell structure and leakage of fluids and protein into the damaged area. The inflammation process begins with increased blood flow and delivery of various substances to the injured area.

These substances include specialized white blood cells, various hormones such as prostaglandins and bradykinins, clotting proteins and more.

The cell damage and resulting inflammation can disrupt the cell's electrical pump and prevent the cell from maintaining its electrical harmony. Oxygen and glucose have a difficult time reaching the injured cells due to defects of the blood flow, and ATP cannot be manufactured. This lack of oxygen to cells (hypoxia) and various irritating chemicals (neurotoxins) signal the nerves to cause pain.

> *In response to the trauma, the soft tissues undergo changes, and the previous pain-free balance in the body is permanently disrupted; post-traumatic fibromyalgia is the outcome.*

In most individuals who have been exposed to trauma, the healing process occurs efficiently and removes damaged cells, rebuilds proteins and tissues, and restores the normal electrical/neurologic balance; and the pain disappears. However, in some individuals who are exposed to the same trauma, there may be a genetic predisposition that destines them to develop post-traumatic fibromyalgia. The trauma "tips the muscles over the edge," so to speak.

What may happen is that the muscles are unable to restore the normal electrical signals. The electrical pumps remain faulty, and various chemicals cause the nerve to remain irritated or sensitized. This in turn creates continuous feedback loops whereby these sensitized nerves send pain signals to the brain. Defects in the muscle blood circulation may not heal, impairing the delivery of oxygen to the area and the removal of irritating waste products from the area. The delivered oxygen to the muscle's energy factory, the mitochondria, may not be used efficiently for manufacture of ATP molecules, causing a lack of energy compounds needed to run the muscle's basic biochemical processes.

As a result of these defective biochemical processes, various muscle fibers can become shortened and develop a state of persistent tension or contraction (localized spasm). This may be how a tender point forms. If certain nerves are sensitized within the tender point and cause referred pain to other areas, a trigger point is present.

> *As a result of these defective biochemical processes following trauma, muscle fibers can become shortened and develop a state of persistent tension or contraction (localized spasm). This may be how a tender point forms.*

These tender and trigger points may be latent; that is, they are present and painful when palpated upon, but do not cause spontaneous pain. Usually, however, these tender and trigger points are spontaneously irritated and cause pain occurring in their particular location, or pain which refers to a different region. These points can be reliably detected upon physical examination, whether they are latent or spontaneously irritated. These tender points usually form where muscle injuries occur but can develop in uninjured muscles as well. Tender points appear to have a predilection for the muscle areas with a high concentration of nerve endings and areas where the muscle inserts into tendon or bone.

Acute muscle injuries will usually heal within six weeks. Some severe soft tissue injuries can take up to four months or longer to heal, but if a soft tissue injury has not healed within six months, and painful tender points are present, then post-traumatic fibromyalgia can be diagnosed.

At the same time the tender points are establishing themselves, other abnormalities may be occurring in post-traumatic fibromyalgia. Various hormonal changes can develop.

1. Serotonin, which helps decrease the central action of pain, becomes low.

2. Growth hormone production decreases.

3. Cortisol has been measured and found to be low in fibromyalgia.

4. Substance P, a small protein hormone called a neurotransmitter, increases to high levels in the spinal fluid, and plays a role in mediating pain from the muscle through the spinal cord and ultimately to the brain.

5. Neuropeptide Y, a product of norepinephrine (another neurotransmitter) decreases in fibromyalgia.

All of these hormonal abnormalities cause specific changes in fibromyalgia.

> *Neurologic abnormalities also develop. The small nerves, particularly the sympathetic nerves, become dysfunctional and may cause feedback loops that create localized muscle spasms and send continuous pain signals to the brain.*

Neurologic abnormalities also develop. The small nerves, particularly the sympathetic nerves, become dysfunctional and may cause feedback loops that create localized muscle spasms and send continuous pain signals to the brain. Sleep-wave abnormalities develop in the brain. This neurologic abnormality prevents normal production of serotonin and growth hormone, which are produced during stage 4 sleep. All hormonal and neurologic changes and abnormalities that occur are closely interrelated in fibromyalgia.

Regional post-traumatic fibromyalgia can turn into generalized post-traumatic fibromyalgia. How might regional pain or regional tender points become more generalized? There may be different mechanisms occurring. A neurologic mechanism occurring at the spinal cord and brain may be a factor. High levels of substance P in the spinal cord at the level where regional muscles were injured may spill over into areas above and below that level and cause pain signals to be transmitted to the brain from levels that were never injured. The entire spine acts as one functional unit, so it is difficult to separate the neck from the lower back. Given that, a localized injury may easily coordinate and synchronize the entire spinal cord pain mechanism to transmit pain signals to the brain, even if the injury involved only one part of the spine.

> *The entire spine acts as one functional unit. Given that, a localized injury may easily coordinate and synchronize the entire spinal cord pain mechanism to transmit pain signals to the brain, even if the injury only involved one part of the spine.*

The dysfunctional sympathetic nerves and decreased serotonin may also play a role in causing abnormal physiologic changes throughout the brain and spinal cord once they are affected by a regional trauma.

Changes in the central nervous system may result from these neurologic and hormonal influences. These changes cause the brain to start recognizing a more widespread pain (generalized post-traumatic fibromyalgia) instead of a localized area of pain (regional post-traumatic fibromyalgia). The central nervous system is sensitized by these neurologic and hormonal changes and begins to sense a more generalized pain. The central nervous system can also send signals back to the muscles to cause continued spasms and tender points in the injured muscles; it can also send signals to uninjured muscle areas and cause tender points to develop.

Individuals who have generalized post-traumatic fibromyalgia who were followed up over time were found to be almost identical to patients who developed primary generalized fibromyalgia. The key difference in this group is the history of trauma that precipitated the condition in the persons with post-traumatic fibromyalgia. Even though we do not know the exact mechanism or cause, the "magic bullet" that ultimately results in the expression of fibromyalgia and post-traumatic fibromyalgia, we know a lot about these conditions and are able to formulate theories about what probably occurs.

All possible theories on the mechanism of post-traumatic fibromyalgia and all abnormalities and their significance are not described in this chapter. Rather, one possible theoretical model based on the key abnormalities is described. With continued research into fibromyalgia, we will better understand the actual pathological mechanism in the cause of fibromyalgia, and perhaps one day discover the single, main pathologic change from which everything else happens, that is, the mythical "magic bullet."

Just as we do not yet know the "magic bullet" cause of fibromyalgia, we do not know the "magic cure." Fibromyalgia is a permanent irreversible condition for which no cure has as yet been discovered.

10

Treatment of Post-Traumatic Fibromyalgia

There is no one single treatment that eliminates symptoms of post-traumatic fibromyalgia. However, various treatments can help individuals with post-traumatic fibromyalgia even if their condition does not disappear or become cured. Each person's treatment program needs to be individualized, and what works for some may not work for others. Hopefully, the patient will find some treatment that is helpful in dealing with the pain.

Following an injury, the patient usually receives a variety of treatments. The treatments that occur immediately after the trauma or within the first few months are called acute treatments. These may include medications, braces, restriction of activity, therapy, or other treatments. For example, the person who sustains an acute whiplash injury following a motor vehicle accident may go to the emergency room and be evaluated and given a cervical collar, which is a soft foam brace to wear around the neck to help support the neck and prevent painful movements. Prescribed medicine may include:

1. An anti-inflammatory drug to reduce pain and swelling

2. A muscle relaxer to decrease muscle spasms

3. Pain medicine to make the patient more comfortable

If the pain persists, the initial treating doctor may order a therapy program which might help decrease some of the pain, at least temporarily. Despite various appropriate acute treatments, the pain persists in people with post-traumatic fibromyalgia.

Whenever treating someone with post-traumatic fibromyalgia, the doctor tries to accomplish specific goals:

- Decreasing pain to a lower, more stable baseline
- Minimizing the flare-ups or exacerbations of the pain
- Improving function, whether it be improving a person's ability to perform job duties, housework, enjoyable hobbies or an exercise program. It is possible to increase function even if the pain does not decrease, but usually decreased pain means better function.
- Finding out what works for the patient, and then getting the patient to carry out a home program on his or her own.

In post-traumatic fibromyalgia various types of treatments are recommended in order to achieve as many individual treatment goals as possible. Some treatments may work better than others, and usually the combination of all the different treatments can lead to overall improvement, even though the post-traumatic fibromyalgia is still present. One of the most important treatment approaches is educating the patient about post-traumatic fibromyalgia.

A person who has chronic pain is often concerned that a life-threatening condition is present. Post-traumatic fibromyalgia causes serious pain, but it is not life-threatening, nor does it turn into another condition, such as rheumatoid arthritis or lupus,

TABLE 4: TREATMENT SUMMARY

Medication	• Analgesics or painkillers • Nonsteroidal anti-inflammatory drugs • Muscle relaxants • Antidepressants • Trigger-point injections/nerve blocks • Miscellaneous
Physical Therapy	• Heat • Whirlpool • Cold • Exercises • Massage • Stretching • Body mechanics • Electric stimulation

Psychological	• Pain and stress management
	• Relaxation techniques
	  - Self-hypnosis
	  - Biofeedback
	• Strategies to deal with:
	  - Fear - Frustration
	  - Anger - Anxiety
	  - Depression

which can cause joint deformities or inflammation. Educating patients about post-traumatic fibromyalgia and reassuring them that they are not going to die from it is an important part of the treatment. Once a person learns about post-traumatic fibromyalgia, he or she can begin to accept this condition and take better control of it.

Medications can be helpful in post-traumatic fibromyalgia. There is no magical pill that will get rid of all fibromyalgia symptoms, but certain drugs can be effective in reducing pain and improving the patient's overall feeling of well-being. No one type of medicine works for everyone and no one medication causes 100% improvement. The patient and doctor often need to experiment with different medicines to find out what works best for any individual. There are various categories of drugs used in the treatment of fibromyalgia:

> *It is up to the individual doctor and patient to formulate strategies for which medicine to use and to assess whether they are working.*

1. **Analgesics or painkillers.** These include over-the-counter medicines such as aspirin, acetaminophen or anti-inflammatories. Prescription-strength medicines can include narcotic medicines and medicines that act on the central nervous system. Pain-relieving ointments, creams and gels that are available over-the-counter can be rubbed into the skin to create a soothing warm or cool sensation that decreases pain.

2. **Nonsteroidal anti-inflammatory drugs (NSAIDs).** This class of medicine is both anti-inflammatory (reduces inflammation) and analgesic (reduces pain). A common drug in this category is ibuprofen, which is available both over-the-counter and by prescription. Because post-traumatic fibromyalgia is not a true inflammation, these drugs may not help much. However, some individuals respond well to these types of medicines, and some that don't respond to this medicine for baseline pain can find it helpful during flare-ups of pain.

3. **Muscle relaxants.** Drugs that cause muscle relaxation can decrease pain in some people. A major side effect of these medications, however, is drowsiness or sedation, and therefore many people do not tolerate these medicines well, including those with post-traumatic fibromyalgia.

4. **Antidepressant medication.** Studies have shown antidepressants can decrease pain in patients with fibromyalgia. In post-traumatic fibromyalgia, two categories of antidepressants, the tricyclic antidepressants and selective serotonin re-uptake inhibitors, can decrease pain, improve sleep and relax muscles.

5. **Trigger-point injections/ nerve blocks.** This treatment is a way of administering medicine, usually a local anesthetic or numbing medicine, directly into the painful tender areas of the muscles or nerves. Trigger-point injections or pain blocks are performed by a doctor who is trained in these techniques.

> *Even if a person has previously undergone physical therapy, I often recommend another course of physical therapy after the patient has been diagnosed with post-traumatic fibromyalgia. Therapy can be more effective if the patient knows the exact diagnosis and understands the treatment rationale.*

There are various other types of medicines that have been used in the treatment of post-traumatic fibromyalgia. It is up to the individual doctor and patient to formulate strategies for which medicines to use and to assess whether they are working.

Physical therapy also often helps. Physical therapies include a wide variety of treatments (heat, cold, massage, electric stimulation, whirlpool, exercises, stretching and more). Even if a person has previously had physical therapy with no benefit, I often recommend another course of physical therapy once the patient been diagnosed with post-traumatic fibromyalgia. Therapy can be more effective if the patient knows the exact diagnosis and understands the treatment rationale of a physical therapy program.

In post-traumatic fibromyalgia, more success is obtained when the emphasis is on teaching a person proper body mechanics and how to avoid positions that aggravate post-traumatic fibromyalgia. These positions include reaching, overhead use of the arms, bending forward, and being in one position for too long. A stretching program and a light conditioning or gentle aerobic program are also important components of therapy in persons with post-traumatic fibromyalgia. These can be learned by the patient and carried out as part of a home program.

> *In chronic post-traumatic fibromyalgia, massotherapy is often the treatment that provides the most relief.*

Massage or massotherapy has been found to be helpful in post-traumatic fibromyalgia. Massage helps decrease pain by several mechanisms, including relaxing muscles, improving circulation and oxygenation, helping remove waste products from the muscles and making the muscles more flexible. In chronic post-traumatic fibromyalgia, massotherapy is often the treatment that provides the most relief.

Osteopathic physicians and chiropractic physicians are trained to perform manipulations and adjustments which can benefit patients with post-traumatic fibromyalgia. These techniques can mobilize joints, improve range of motion, relax muscles and reduce muscle pain.

Manipulations are forceful movements of body parts such as the neck to bring about a greater range of motion and relax muscles. Adjustments are the application of a specific and precise force to a specific point in the vertebrae or muscle to properly align the body. The desired outcome is improved circulation and neurologic flow, which reduce tension and pain.

Since post-traumatic fibromyalgia involves the entire person, mind and muscles, not just the muscles, a successful treatment approach usually involves helping persons mentally manage their fibromyalgia pain. Chronic physical pain will ultimately cause psychological reactions including fear, frustration, anger, anxiety and even depression. Psychological stress can interfere with a person's self-esteem and interpersonal relationships, and affect one's entire lifestyle.

> **Counseling can help an individual overcome feelings of depression and frustration brought on by chronic pain associated with post-traumatic fibromyalgia.**

Mentally managing fibromyalgia can involve treatment approaches that include working with a psychologist or counselor for pain and stress management, or learning relaxation techniques through self-hypnosis, biofeedback or self-awareness. Biofeedback is a technique in which individuals learn to control their bodily responses to achieve relaxation and pain relief. Psychotherapy and counseling can help an individual overcome feelings of depression and frustration brought on by chronic pain.

Treatment approaches for chronic pain include traditional medicine approaches and alternative medicine approaches. Perhaps the best outcomes are obtained when a knowledgeable doctor combines the best of both traditional and alternative medicines and formulates a successful individualized treatment program for the person with post-traumatic fibromyalgia.

There are several possible responses to treatments of post-traumatic fibromyalgia:

1. The person feels better.
2. The person feels worse.
3. The person feels the same.

Measuring one's response to treatment involves subjective responses (what the patient says happens as a result of the treatment), as well as objective responses (what can be measured on examination as a result of the treatments or in response to the treatments).

If a person receiving treatment reports improvement, I usually ask him or her to quantitate the improvement. The person may express a percentage of improvement from the original pain, or use a numbering system on a 0 to 10 scale, with 0 being no pain and 10 being the worst pain. An example of an improved response is the patient reporting 40% improvement overall in terms of decreased pain, with the pain ranging from 3 to 6 out of 10 where it used to be 6 to 10 out of 10.

> **Since post-traumatic fibromyalgia is a chronic and permanent condition, invariably there will be a medical need for future treatments.**

Many times the patient reports that physical therapies and other treatments help temporarily, but that within a few hours or days the pain returns to its original higher level. Others may report no substantial improvement in pain, but they feel more flexible and have more motion and movement in their joints and muscles. Occasionally, individuals will report no improvement whatsoever with any of the treatments and may even state that certain types of treatments such as attempted exercises and physical therapy have aggravated the pain.

The doctor tries to characterize the responses to all these treatments during follow-up examinations. What the doctor is actually doing is taking another history, an interim history between the last visit and current visit, and determining current symptoms and nature of the pain. An interim physical examination will be performed to determine abnormal physical findings and to note any changes that may indicate objective improvement to a specific treatment program.

Characterization of the tender points is part of the follow-up physical exam. Are the tender points less painful, less tense, or smaller in size? Are there more tender points, or fewer bothersome tender points? Tender points may become less painful during treatment and the patient will indicate less "spontaneous" pain in a certain region, even though, upon palpation, the painful tender points will still be present.

Certainly a goal of treatment is to make tender points go into remission. This happens when tender points go from being spontaneously painful to being latent or quiet tender points. Upon palpation of these latent tender points, the pain is still present so the tender points have not "disappeared."

> *If a person benefits from any type of treatment, even if only temporarily, the patient and doctor may determine that this temporary response improves the person's quality of life. For this reason, it is medically necessary to continue with these treatments.*

Follow-up physical examinations include measurement of localized muscle spasms, which will usually decrease in patients who have improved. Range of motion of the neck, back or shoulders can also show improvement if the patient is having successful results with a treatment program.

In evaluating an individual person's response to a treatment program, the doctor must determine what the need for future treatments will be. Since post-traumatic fibromyalgia is a chronic and permanent condition, invariably there will be a medical need for future treatments. This issue is discussed more fully in Chapter 11.

A person with post-traumatic fibromyalgia may require an ongoing maintenance or supportive therapy program to keep the pain under control and allow improved functioning in his or her everyday life. Quality of life issues are looked at when future treatments are determined. If a person benefits from any type of treatment, even if only temporarily, the patient and doctor may determine that this temporary response improves the person's quality of life. For this reason, it is medically necessary to continue with these treatments.

> *I do not encourage ongoing, indefinite supervised medical treatment. Rather, I promote individual responsibility for following through with an independent, unsupervised home program to control the chronic problems associated with fibromyalgia.*

A program that includes periodic doctor follow-ups, medications, and a home program (heat, stretching, light conditioning) is often recommended. I try to get patients on an independent home program that is successful for them even though they still have a baseline level of pain. However, flare-ups are expected with fibromyalgia. A flare-up may occur that causes pain which the patient is not able to control on his or her own with the home program. In such cases, an additional physical therapy program or other type of supervised medical program may be required in order to help the individual achieve a stable baseline level of pain again.

The medical necessity of any treatment program is determined for each individual by the doctor. Treatments are not recommended or continued if they have no effect on patients. If treatments are deemed helpful, they are continued as long as they help or until a patient learns an independent home program that is effective and reduces the need for professionally supervised treatments.

I do not encourage ongoing, indefinite supervised medical treatment. Rather, I promote individual responsibility for following through with an independent, unsupervised home program to control the chronic problems associated with fibromyalgia.

11

Prognosis In Post-Traumatic Fibromyalgia

Prognosis is defined as a forecast of the probable outcome of a condition. Doctors try to determine whether there will be recovery by studying the nature and particular features of the medical condition. Determining a prognosis is one of the most important yet difficult aspects in the practice of medicine. A physician's knowledge of an individual's conditions, symptoms and physical findings and natural progression of the pain, combined with his or her experience in treating individuals with a particular condition, is important in determining any given prognosis. In medicolegal terms, the prognosis is a medical forecast based on the probability that it is more likely than not that a particular outcome will occur.

Post-traumatic fibromyalgia is a chronic and permanent condition. Once this condition has developed and is clinically measurable upon examination, it will be present for the remainder of the person's life. In all of the literature on fibromyalgia, based on clinical experience and discussion among various doctors who treat fibromyalgia, I am aware of no cure for fibromyalgia (or post-traumatic fibromyalgia). We hope that one day there will be a cure, but the present reality is that post-traumatic fibromyalgia is an incurable disorder.

The symptoms of post-traumatic fibromyalgia can improve. There may be less pain over time. The condition can go from being severely painful to minimally painful, but it is still there. Post-traumatic fibromyalgia, despite improvement or lessening of the overall condition, never disappears. Thus, a complete recovery is impossible with post-traumatic fibromyalgia. This is the same as saying 100% healing does not occur, but healing can occur, and it always does so at a final percentage of less than 100%.

> *In medicolegal terms, the prognosis is a medical forecast based on the probability that it is more likely than not that a particular outcome will occur.*

Follow-up studies on individuals with post-traumatic fibromyalgia done by doctors (including Dr. Waylonis and Dr. Romano) have shown that post-traumatic fibromyalgia continued to be present years after the initial diagnosis. Furthermore, the vast majority of these patients continued to require treatment. If litigation was involved, individuals continued to have post-traumatic fibromyalgia and require treatment even after settlement of the litigation.

If post-traumatic fibromyalgia is incurable, what can be expected over time for these individuals? Post-traumatic fibromyalgia causes pain, mainly, and therefore individuals will have a baseline level of pain. Some people will have high levels of pain, whereas others may have minimal baseline levels of pain.

Flare-ups are expected periodically in these individuals as part of the natural long-term course of post-traumatic fibromyalgia. Flare-ups are an aggravation or an exacerbation of the baseline level of pain and usually are temporary, lasting from days to weeks before the pain returns to the previous stable baseline.

There are a variety of reasons why an individual will experience a flare-up of post-traumatic fibromyalgia:

- Certain physical activities, particularly too much activity, can cause a flare-up.
- Too little activity can also aggravate symptoms. Muscles in fibromyalgia require a baseline level of exercise, and any level of activity below this baseline threshold can cause flare-ups.
- Viral syndromes or the flu can lead to flare-ups.
- Women may notice a flare-up of symptoms related to the fluid-retention stage of the menstrual cycle.
- Cold, damp conditions and drafts can cause flare-ups.
- Emotional stress plays a role in flare-ups.

> *The vast majority of these patients continue to require treatment. If litigation was involved, individuals continued to have post-traumatic fibromyalgia and require treatment even after settlement of the litigation.*

Perhaps the most common cause of post-traumatic fibromyalgia flare-ups is "unknown cause." A flare-up may be unrelated to any physical, environmental, psychosocial factor; the pain simply spontaneously increases. Flare-ups are a part of post-traumatic fibromyalgia so they are not to be considered unusual or a complication of post-traumatic fibromyalgia.

Although we know flare-ups will occur, we cannot predict exactly when or how frequently they will occur. Upon review of my own patients with post-traumatic fibromyalgia, I note that persons have an average of two major flare-ups per year. A major flare-up is defined as increased regional or generalized pain when compared to a stable baseline level, that persists for at least three consecutive days and interferes with usual daily activities. The average duration of each flare-up is one month. These figures were determined by a retrospective review of patients, but there was wide disparity among individual patients.

By following individual patients over a period of time, we can reasonably predict how many flare-ups they will have over the next year based on how many flare-ups they've averaged over preceding years. However, we have no way of determining the frequency of flare-ups in a patient newly diagnosed with post-traumatic fibromyalgia.

> *From a medical standpoint, limitations or restrictions are necessary in post-traumatic fibromyalgia. These limitations give physical guidelines on what the person can and cannot do to minimize the chances of an exacerbation.*

Post-traumatic fibromyalgia causes limitations in a person's function or abilities. These limitations may affect basic activities involved in daily living, activities around the home or activities at work.

Post-traumatic fibromyalgia causes individuals to complain of difficulty performing activities that involve a lot of reaching or outstretched use of the arms such as housecleaning, running a vacuum, painting or working on an assembly line. Being in one position for too long, whether it be standing or sitting, usually causes pain and interferes with tasks such as school classes, typing or working on the job. People complain about pain and fatigue when working a normal work-day or when performing tasks that require several hours or more, to the point where they may be unable to finish these activities.

Patients with post-traumatic fibromyalgia are more likely to complain of limitations that result in loss of employment, reduced physical activity, inability to pursue previously enjoyed hobbies or recreational activities, or receiving disability compensation. Post-traumatic fibromyalgia frequently results in inability to perform usual job duties because of pain and associated impairment.

From a medical standpoint, limitations or restrictions are necessary in post-traumatic fibromyalgia.

These limitations give physical guidelines on what the person can and cannot do to minimize the chances of an exacerbation.

Examples of work restrictions specific to a person with post-traumatic fibromyalgia might include:

1. No working more than eight hours a day, five days a week. Specifically, no overtime or weekends

2. Working part-time hours, or working day hours only; or working flexible hours

3. Avoiding temperature changes (no exposure to cold, damp weather)

> *Post-traumatic fibromyalgia causes pain and limitations of functional abilities, but that doesn't mean that a person will become completely and totally disabled. In fact, total and permanent disability occurs infrequently in people with post-traumatic fibromyalgia.*

4. No exposure to direct air-conditioning drafts

5. No repetitive reaching or overhead use of the arms

6. No repetitive bending or leaning forward

7. No sitting, standing or walking for a long time before alternating between positions

Disability issues frequently arise in post-traumatic fibromyalgia and they need to be handled on an individual basis between the patient and the doctor. Post-traumatic fibromyalgia causes pain and limitations of functional abilities as described, but that doesn't mean that a person will become completely and totally disabled. In fact, total and permanent disability occurs infrequently in people with post-traumatic fibromyalgia. The majority of persons, however, have some type of disability as a result of post-traumatic fibromyalgia.

In understanding disabilities, we need to explain some definitions. The World Health Organization has developed the following definitions:

Impairment. Any loss or abnormality of psychological, physical or anatomical structure or function. In post-traumatic fibromyalgia, 100% of people will have some impairment, by definition, because the tender points are considered an impairment.

Disability. Any restriction or lack of an ability to perform an activity in the manner or within the range considered normal for a human being. It is possible for someone with very mild post-traumatic fibromyalgia to have an impairment without a disability, but the vast majority of people with post-traumatic fibromyalgia will have some type of disability or restriction as described above. These restrictions, such as the inability to perform repetitive reaching, bending, twisting or standing, are considered permanent restrictions and therefore a permanent disability.

Disability can be further categorized into partial or total, particularly when used in the occupational setting. An individual with total disability has restrictions that prevent him or her from performing any type of employment. An individual with partial disability will have restrictions interfering with certain job activities but is capable to perform some type of job activities within these restrictions.

Handicap. A disadvantage for a given individual resulting from an impairment or disability that limits or prevents the fulfillment of a role that is normal for that individual. This role depends on age, gender, and social and cultural factors. Individuals with post-traumatic fibromyalgia who ultimately lose their jobs, receive disability compensation, have break-ups of personal relationships or other problems, are handicapped because of post-traumatic fibromyalgia.

These definitions can be cumbersome in the clinical practice when pertaining to post-traumatic fibromyalgia. When we speak in terms of prognosis, all individuals with post-traumatic fibromyalgia have some type of impairment, and nearly all have a disability. The probability is high as well that any individual with post-traumatic fibromyalgia, over time, will become handicapped as a result of this condition. The ultimate recognition and determination of an individual's particular consequences are the responsibility of the treating physician.

> *All individuals with post-traumatic fibromyalgia have some type of impairment, and nearly all have a disability. The probability is high as well that any individual with post-traumatic fibromyalgia, over time, will become handicapped as a result of this condition.*

Part of the prognosis includes determining medical necessity of future treatments in post-traumatic fibromyalgia. Again, any individual's future course cannot be exactly determined, but we can speak in terms of probabilities or opinions based on reasonable medical certainty. Because post-traumatic fibromyalgia is a chronic and permanent condition, causing limitations characterized by a baseline level of pain with periodic flare-ups, it is probable that the individual will require future treatments. They would include:

1. Periodic doctor visits

2. Medications, whether they be prescription or over-the-counter, or a combination

3. Therapies, whether they be adjustments, modalities, a supervised physical therapy program, or a home program of stretching and exercise

4. Activity modifications that could include restricted job hours, restricted activities, or increased rest

Because flare-ups occur, medically necessary supervised treatments will usually be required if the flare-up overwhelms the person's ability to effectively use a home program to control the pain. A follow-up evaluation by the treating physician and prescription of an appropriate treatment program are required for the individual's flare-ups.

> **Because flare-ups occur, medically necessary supervised treatments will usually be required if the flare-up overwhelms the person's ability to effectively use a home program to control the pain.**

Individuals with post-traumatic fibromyalgia are at risk for developing other associated conditions. As indicated in Chapter 9, regional post-traumatic fibromyalgia can turn into a more generalized form over time. Other associated conditions, including anxiety disorder, sleep disorder, irritable bowel syndrome, fatigue and depression, can develop over time. People with post-traumatic fibromyalgia may be at risk of developing accelerated degenerative arthritis or osteoarthritis over time. This arthritic condition can lead to further pain, limitation of joint motion and damage to nerve roots or the spinal cord.

Unfortunately, the future of patients with post-traumatic fibromyalgia is not favorable. Life expectancy is not affected by fibromyalgia, nor are patients destined to live a poor quality life or become totally disabled. But patients will continue to have pain, flare-ups and functional limitations that interfere with their future and usually require medical intervention.

2. The patient's characterization of increased pain

3. The exam findings of new tender points

4. The need for more treatment since the trauma.

Pre-Existing Associated Conditions

Many individuals with post-traumatic fibromyalgia will have a history of one or more of the associated conditions seen with fibromyalgia prior to the actual trauma. Associated conditions seen with fibromyalgia include allergies, anxiety disorders, depression, headaches, irritable bowel syndrome, jaw joint (TMJ) dysfunction, fatigue and sleep problems.

The presence of one or more of these conditions does not indicate the presence of fibromyalgia, however. That is like putting the cart before the horse. One needs to have chronic pain with a characteristic pattern of tender points to have a diagnosis of fibromyalgia. Without these key features of fibromyalgia, none of the associated conditions by themselves, or in combination, carries any significant meaning when determining the presence of fibromyalgia. These associated conditions follow fibromyalgia as the cart follows the horse. And the horse (fibromyalgia) needs to be present and pulling the cart (associated conditions).

The presence of one or more associated conditions may increase the risk of an individual eventually developing fibromyalgia. However, many people without fibromyalgia have one or more of these common associated conditions. Some of these people may develop fibromyalgia over time, but

12

Special Situations in Post-Traumatic Fibromyalgia

Post-traumatic fibromyalgia is usually a direct consequence of a single trauma. By this I mean that the individual had no previous pain problems until a trauma, then developed post-traumatic fibromyalgia after the trauma. No other pain problems existed before the injury, at the time of the injury, or following the injury. However, not all patients will follow this "straightforward" course. There are special situations that involve post-traumatic fibromyalgia that will be addressed in this chapter.

There are several categories of special situations in post-traumatic fibromyalgia. The first category involves problems that pre-dated the trauma. Examples in this category would be the presence of fibromyalgia in individuals before a trauma, or the presence of associated conditions seen with fibromyalgia, such as depression, irritable bowel syndrome or headaches, before the trauma.

Another category involves problems that occurred at the time of injury in addition to the injuries that led to post-traumatic fibromyalgia. Trauma victims frequently suffer such additional problems or injuries as closed head injury or concussion, bone fracture, herniated disk, or a tendon/ligament rupture.

The third category involves additional problems that occur after the injury that caused post-traumatic fibromyalgia. In this category, depression, chronic pain syndrome, additional traumas, and malingering are included.

Pre-Existing Fibromyalgia

The key points of the history in an individual with fibromyalgia and a new trauma are to determine if there are new areas of pain that did not exist before the trauma, and if the pain is more severe.

In a person who has pre-existing fibromyalgia before being involved in a particular trauma, it is important to determine what was the baseline level prior to the trauma. Included in the history of the baseline level would be the location and severity of the pain and what activities could or could not be performed. The doctor would need to know what medical treatments were required for the fibromyalgia prior to the trauma, how often was the treatment needed, when was the last treatment before the trauma, and what were previous documentations of the physical exam?

Just as trauma can cause the development of post-traumatic fibromyalgia from a previous baseline of "no pain," so can this same trauma cause an increase in pain when compared to a previous baseline of "some" pain.

There are two things that can happen when a person with fibromyalgia sustains a trauma. Either there is no overall worsening of the fibromyalgia with the trauma, or there is worsening of the pain with the trauma. I have never encountered anyone who reported improvement of pain following a trauma. Usually, the pain is worsened. In those whose pain becomes worse, several things can happen over time: The pain improves, the pain stays the same, or the pain gets worse. The level of pain may return to the previous baseline, or it may stay permanently above this previous baseline.

Of key importance in a
fibromyalgia and a new traum
there are new areas of pain that
ously and if the pain is more
ments that were given since the
reviewed to determine whether
they helped or not. Any change
in activity (for example, time off
from work or inability to work)
needs to be documented.

The physical exam will determine if tender points are present
in new locations. Reviewing
records of previous physical exams can determine if new tender points are present in different locations since the trauma.

Just as one must wait six months
after an injury before the presence of pos
fibromyalgia can be verified as a chroni
manent condition, one must also wait si
following a trauma superimposed on pre
fibromyalgia before permanent worsenin
baseline level of pain can be determined.

If the pain improves to the previous stabl
line, then the increased pain caused by the
is considered a temporary condition. That
trauma caused a temporary flare-up of fibro
gia that resolved with no permanent worse
However, if the pain remains higher than the p
ous baseline after six months, then one may
clude that the trauma has caused a permanent w
ening of the previous stable fibromyalgia.
conclusion of permanent worsening is based o
combination of factors:

1. Passage of six months time from the trauma

Associated
with fibrom
lergies, anx
pression, h
bowel syr
function,
problems.
any of the
not indica
bromyalg

others may not. Ongoing research may ultimately show that individuals with certain pre-existing associated conditions are more at risk for developing fibromyalgia following a trauma, compared to a group of people without the pre-existing conditions exposed to a similar trauma. I believe, however, that these studies will also show that the key cause of the actual fibromyalgia condition was the trauma itself.

Additional Injuries Other Than Post-Traumatic Fibromyalgia

Trauma can cause various tissue injuries in addition to muscle and soft tissue injuries that ultimately lead to post-traumatic fibromyalgia. Examples of these additional injuries include:

1. **Closed head injury/concussion.** If the head is struck, brain injury can occur. There may be loss of consciousness. Individuals with head injuries may develop a condition called **post-concussive syndrome,** which is a lingering condition following concussion that causes ongoing problems. The patient complaints include:

   - Headaches
   - Dizziness
   - Fatigue
   - Irritability
   - Insomnia
   - Poor coordination
   - Depression
   - Anxiety
   - Problems with hearing, vision, and smell
   - Sensitivity to loud noises, bright lights and crowds
   - Difficulty with memory and concentration

   Standardized memory and personality testing may reveal problems in these areas specific to head injury. This condition is separate from post-traumatic fibromyalgia, but it has many overlapping symptoms.

2. Herniated disk. Spinal injuries can lead to rupture of the disk between the vertebrae. This ruptured disk can cause pressure and inflammation of the spinal cord or nerve roots and lead to loss of reflexes, sensation abnormality, weakness or paralysis. This condition may require a specific therapy program or even surgery to remove the herniated disk. Lingering pain problems can occur from scar tissue, damaged nerves, vertebral imbalances or spinal arthritis. These residual pain problems may overlap with the pain in post-traumatic fibromyalgia.

> *If the doctor feels that the pain is coming from both post-traumatic fibromyalgia and residuals from another condition, he or she tries to determine what percentage of pain is coming from one versus the other.*

3. Bone fractures. During acute trauma, bones may fracture. Fractures can occur in the spinal column, in the long bones or at the joints. Fracture treatments include immobilization, casting or surgical repairs. The fractures usually heal completely, but sometimes residual pain syndromes can result due to the bony injury, post-traumatic arthritis or nerve injuries.

Various other associated injuries can occur at the time of the trauma. The challenge to the doctor who is examining the patient over time is to determine which residual symptoms, particularly pain, are attributed to post-traumatic fibromyalgia and which to residual result of these other injuries. If the doctor feels that the pain is coming from both post-traumatic fibromyalgia and residuals from another condition, he or she tries to determine what percentage of pain is coming from one versus the other. The doctor may determine that only post-traumatic fibromyalgia is causing the pain and that the other injuries have completely healed and are pain-free or asymptomatic.

Additional Problems That Develop After Trauma

Once post-traumatic fibromyalgia develops, the person is at risk for developing the associated conditions previously mentioned. Forty to fifty percent of people with fibromyalgia will develop depression. Other associated conditions that commonly develop include fatigue, headaches and irritable bowel syndrome. People may initially have a regional post-traumatic fibromyalgia but over the course of time develop additional tender points even in areas that were not injured, and ultimately have generalized post-traumatic fibromyalgia.

The doctor needs to determine if additional conditions have developed, and what is each condition's contribution to the patient's overall clinical picture. Associated conditions may require separate intensive treatment programs altogether. For example, depression may require treatment with antidepressant medicine, psychological counseling, or a referral to a psychiatrist. Irritable bowel syndrome may require gastrointestinal testing or a specialized evaluation by a gastroenterologist.

There are some special situations that can occur after the injury. These include:

1. **A subsequent trauma** in addition to the original trauma. A patient with a second trauma that occurs after the original trauma has caused post-traumatic fibromyalgia needs to be handled in the same way as an individual with pre-existing fibromyalgia who undergoes trauma.

   The baseline following the first trauma needs to be determined, and any new problems associated with the second trauma need to be carefully reviewed. New areas of pain, new functional limitations, new associated symptoms and new physical findings all need to be determined. The question that needs to be addressed is: Is there increased pain that is considered a temporary flare-up, or has there been permanent worsening from a previous stable baseline as a result of the additional trauma?

2. Chronic Pain Syndrome. Some individuals with post-traumatic fibromyalgia develop a condition known as chronic pain syndrome. This is defined as a state of overwhelming chronic pain that interferes with the person's physical, emotional and psychological functional abilities and causes disruption in everyday life activities. Characteristics of a person with chronic pain include:

> *Chronic pain syndrome is defined as a state of overwhelming chronic pain that interferes with the person's physical, emotional and psychological functional abilities and causes disruption in everyday life activities.*

a. **Significant subjective and functional limitations that are out of proportion** to the objective physical exam findings

b. **Dependency and addictive behaviors** (excessive medicines, alcohol, nicotine, etc.)

c. **Well-defined pain behaviors.** Examples of pain behaviors include slow, deliberate movements, walking with an inconsistent limp, exaggerated flinching upon palpation, frequent facial grimacing and sighing, and frequent indication of "I can't" when asked to perform a certain movement or physical task.

The person who has developed chronic pain syndrome will give a history of terrible pain for which nothing has helped and everything has been tried, but the condition continues to get worse. The patient will report that he or she cannot do anything and may spend most of the time in bed. These patients often complain of feeling depressed, frustrated and anxious, and describe themselves as disabled.

Typically the physical examination is very difficult with these patients because of the pain behaviors. There is usually exaggerated pain responses including flinching, facial grimacing, crying out or complaining of pain with light palpation in any area.

> *The examiner may conclude that the patient is probably able to do more he or she indicates or attempts. Thus, a patient's subjective limitations are out of proportion to the examiner's objective findings.*

Neurologic testing, particularly sensory testing and muscle strength testing, may be impossible because the patient is not able to cooperate in a reliable manner. Likewise, attempting to localize specific painful tender points can be very difficult if the patient is complaining of pain wherever he or she is touched. The examiner may conclude that the patient is probably able to do more than he or she indicates or attempts. Thus, a patient's subjective limitations are out of proportion to the examiner's objective findings.

The person with chronic pain syndrome does have true pain. A psychological reaction to this chronic pain, however, has led to the diagnosis of the chronic pain syndrome as described above. The medical examiner is challenged to "isolate" post-traumatic fibromyalgia in the presence of the overall chronic pain syndrome. Post-traumatic fibromyalgia is a painful condition, but it usually does not develop into chronic pain syndrome. When it does, both conditions, chronic pain syndrome and post-traumatic fibromyalgia, are considered consequences of the original trauma. Post-traumatic fibromyalgia occurs first, and then chronic pain syndrome develops.

Malingering

> *The person with chronic pain syndrome does have true pain. A psychological reaction to this chronic pain, however, has led to the diagnosis of the chronic pain syndrome.*

In my experience, a true malingerer is rare. Chronic pain syndrome is more common and is not to be misinterpreted as malingering. In chronic pain syndrome, the mechanisms are subconscious; that is, the person has no conscious "input" into this condition's development. A malingerer is one who willfully, deliberately and fraudulently creates or exaggerates symptoms of an illness or injury for the purpose of a consciously desired end result. This desired end result may include a financial settlement, disability, medications or something else. Because a lot has been written in detail about fibromyalgia, there is a potential risk that a deceitful individual can read and learn about fibromyalgia and attempt to deceive a medical examiner.

There are various techniques that medical doctors use to spot the malingerer. Inconsistencies in the history, or the history that is "too perfect," should be a red flag that the person may be malingering. Clinical intuition often comes into play in suspecting a person to be a malingerer.

The physical examination can reveal discrepancies. Inconsistent patterns of tender points that are not reproducible, tender points that are in incorrect locations, and the absence of localized spasms should alert the physician to a possible malingerer. Two techniques can be used during the physical exam. One is distracting the patient to a certain region while palpating a different body region to look for reproducible tender points. A true tender point will be painful whether the person is focusing on this area or is distracted from the area during the palpation. Another technique is to focus on an area that would not be expected to be a tender point, and observing the patient response.

Areas that receive intense focus by the physician can often trigger a malingerer to attempt to feign an abnormal finding in that area.

All inconsistent findings and observations need to be carefully documented, and the physician needs to indicate in the diagnostic impression that he or she does not feel a serious medical problem exists, i.e., no posttraumatic fibromyalgia, and

Chronic pain syndrome is not to be misinterpreted as malingering. In chronic pain syndrome, the mechanisms are subconscious. A malingerer is one who deliberately creates or exaggerates symptoms for the purpose of a consciously desired end result (a financial settlement, disability or medications).

that the person appears to be malingering. I believe a true malingerer is rare and that a malingerer who can fool a knowledgeable physician is even rarer.

13

Who Is a Fibromyalgia Expert?

Even though fibromyalgia has been described in multiple medical and consumer journals, and hundreds of research articles have appeared in the last decade, not everyone recognizes fibromyalgia as a legitimate medical syndrome. As discussed in Chapter 2, reputable medical doctors have stated that fibromyalgia does not exist. This statement, however, represents an uninformed medical opinion. Medical opinions about a particular condition are as abundant as doctors, and some opinions are based on scientific knowledge and fact, whereas others are based on personal biases.

Certain criteria should be acknowledged in determining who is knowledgeable about fibromyalgia and able to provide a credible opinion. Not everyone can be an expert in fibromyalgia, even if the person is a physician. The criteria in determining who is a fibromyalgia expert include training, research background, clinical experience, personal experience, ongoing education, and peer opinion.

Training

A physician whose specialty involved neuro-musculoskeletal training will usually learn about fibromyalgia and how to palpate tender points and make a diagnosis of fibromyalgia or post-traumatic fibromyalgia. Two specialties in particular, physical medicine and rehabilitation, and rheumatology, receive more focused training on muscle disorders such as fibromyalgia. Most orthopedic specialties also provide good training in evaluating and diagnosing muscular disorders such as fibromyalgia. Fibromyalgia fellowships have been offered in some specialized residency programs that include one year of specialized fibromyalgia training. Specialty training, a fellowship, intensive preceptorship, or a specialized chiropractic program may enable a doctor to acquire adequate knowledge and experience to qualify him or her as a fibromyalgia expert.

Research Background

Doctors who design research projects and publish them in medical journals acquire considerable knowledge and skills in fibromyalgia. Research projects involve a lot of time, planning, evaluation of people, review of results, and preparation of the research article. All of this exposes the individual to current scientific knowledge of fibromyalgia, including works published by other authors. Most of the leading fibromyalgia experts today are also leading researchers.

Clinical Experience

Understanding and diagnosing fibromyalgia require exposure to patients. A doctor who has treated numerous patients with fibromyalgia over a period of time will gain valuable training and experience in this condition. The doctor will become skillful with the tender point examination and learn to appreciate subtle abnormalities in muscle tissues by palpation.

The doctor who sees few fibromyalgia patients will

> *Understanding and diagnosing fibromyalgia require exposure to patients. A doctor who has treated numerous fibromyalgia patients gains valuable experience in the tender point examination and learns to appreciate very subtle abnormalities in muscle tissues by palpation.*

not have the opportunity to practice and perfect the physical examination of the tender points and will not acquire expertise in fibromyalgia. Most fibromyalgia experts have diagnosed and treated thousands of fibromyalgia patients.

Personal Experience

As a physician with fibromyalgia, I have a unique opportunity to understand how fibromyalgia affects an individual. Any medical professional who has a personal perspective on a particular condition will certainly become more knowledgeable and experienced in diag-

Recent research in the field of fibromyalgia has led to evolution in opinions and treatment strategies. Doctors who treat patients with fibromyalgia need to maintain current knowledge of scientific research.

nosing and treating this disorder by bridging personal and professional experiences.

Ongoing Education

Doctors need to continue to learn after their residency training program. A lot of research has taken place in recent years in the field of fibromyalgia. Opinions have evolved and treatment strategies have changed. Doctors who treat patients with fibromyalgia need to maintain current knowledge of scientific research. Ways to maintain current knowledge include attending seminars or conferences, reading the medical journals and accessing computer data banks on fibromyalgia.

Peer Opinion

Probably the most credible opinions regarding a given doctor's abilities are those provided by that doctor's peers. If experts in a particular field consider another doctor to be a qualified expert as well in that field, then the highest standards are being met. Individuals who have achieved a high standard of expertise in fibromyalgia will apply those same standards to another individual before considering that doctor an expert as well.

A fibromyalgia expert would be one that meets one or more of these criteria, with the most important criterion being the "peer opinion." An individual who meets none of the above criteria should not be regarded as a fibromyalgia expert.

> *Expertise in fibromyalgia is critical to one who provides medicolegal opinions or testimony involving fibromyalgia. A fibromyalgia expert will be able to provide very specific information about fibromyalgia that is considered credible, reliable and scientifically correct.*

A doctor does not have to be a fibromyalgia expert to be able to diagnose and treat a person with fibromyalgia and provide competent, compassionate care. The issue of being a fibromyalgia expert is critical, however, to one who provides medicolegal opinions or testimony involving fibromyalgia. A fibromyalgia expert will be able to provide very specific information about fibromyalgia that is considered credible, reliable, and scientifically correct.

14

Medical Testimony In Post-Traumatic Fibromyalgia

Many times, individuals with post-traumatic fibromyalgia find themselves involved in litigation. Fibromyalgia is a medical condition that has been recognized by the federal government, Worker's Compensation, Social Security and the courts.

This recognition does not necessarily mean automatic reimbursement in the litigation setting. Financial settlements have varied from very little to large amounts. The determining difference is usually how convincingly one side or the other presents its case to the judge or jury regarding pain and suffering from post-traumatic fibromyalgia.

Various percentages of disability have been awarded by the Social Security and Worker's Compensation systems, with wide variations occurring among regions, states and doctors. Individuals with post-traumatic fibromyalgia often accumulate extensive medical bills, and if these medical costs are not reimbursed by an insurance company, then a personal injury lawsuit may be filed that could ultimately end up in court.

From the patient's perspective, the litigation process is very stressful, and stress is known to aggravate post-traumatic fibromyalgia symptoms. Mental stress is not the cause of post-traumatic fibromyalgia, but it can definitely be a factor in a flare-up, particularly during legal proceedings. These proceedings are inherently stressful to the person due to time involved and the dominance of the patient's life by the multiple issues. The majority of my patients report significant reduction of stress once the litigation issue has been settled.

The physician treating fibromyalgia may be asked to provide medical testimony at times. There are various ways that medical testimony can be provided:

- A narrative medical report detailing specific diagnosis, treatments and prognosis can be generated for the attorney.
- Videotape depositions or live testimony in court can be presented.

I have frequently been asked to provide medical testimony in various fashions, most commonly preparing a narrative medical report for the attorney. Often I will be asked to provide a videotaped deposition, and occasionally I have given live testimony in court.

As a doctor who treats fibromyalgia, I am usually requested to provide medical testimony on behalf of my patient, the plaintiff. I have provided medical testimony for defense attorneys as well.

As a medical witness, I am commonly asked questions from the defense attorney regarding post-traumatic fibromyalgia. I have summarized some of the most common questions asked of me and how I answer them.

1. How could a serious injury have resulted when there was only minor damage to the car?

ANSWER: There is usually no correlation between the severity of the injury and how much damage was done to the car. Severe neck injuries have been described during collisions occurring when the offending car was moving less than 10 miles per hour. Minor vehicle impacts can still create damaging forces to body tissues such as muscles.

2. How could a serious condition be present if all the tests and X-rays were normal?

ANSWER: There is no specific test or X-ray that detects fibromyalgia. Therefore, laboratory tests and X-rays are **expected** to be normal because they are looking for conditions other than fibromyalgia. In a serious condition such as fibromyalgia, one would expect all the routine tests and X-rays to be normal; otherwise, a condition other than fibromyalgia is present.

3. Could the person have developed fibromyalgia even if there was no injury?

ANSWER: Many individuals develop fibromyalgia. It is a common condition occurring in 2%-5% of the population. Some people are more vulnerable to developing fibromyalgia, probably due to genetic factors, but it is not possible to predict what given individual will develop fibromyalgia over the course of his or her lifetime.

People who develop fibromyalgia in the absence of any injury usually do so in a gradual fashion. That is, the muscle pain begins gradually and worsens over a period of months and years until ultimately a diagnosis of fibromyalgia is made.

A person who develops fibromyalgia after an injury, however, develops **immediate severe pain** at the time of the injury, and **this pain persists indefinitely** as part of post-traumatic fibromyalgia.

In an individual who has post-traumatic fibromyalgia, the probability is very low that this individual would have ever developed acute spontaneous fibromyalgia on a particular date had there been no injury on that particular date.

4. If the cause of fibromyalgia is not known, how can we be certain that trauma causes it?

ANSWER: Although we do not know the exact pathologic mechanism or sequence of events that leads to fibromyalgia, we know of various causes of fibromyalgia, including trauma.

There is a difference between a known cause of a medical condition and the exact mechanism of how this medical condition develops. For example, we knew that cigarette smoking caused lung cancer years before we knew the exact way that it led to lung cancer. Many medical conditions have known causes but still-unexplained exact mechanisms. We know a lot about the abnormalities in fibromyalgia, but we still do not know the exact pathological changes that occur from the trauma that lead to fibromyalgia.

5. Since the person needs to indicate pain during the tender point examination, are the tender points considered a subjective and not objective finding?

ANSWER: Tender points are considered objective findings, requiring a knowledgeable physician to detect them. Tender points are distinct soft tissue areas that usually have a peculiar abnormal consistency to them.

Although the patient reports pain during the tender point exam, there are other requirements for positive painful tender points. They include the ability to reproduce or redemonstrate those tender points by palpation, finding the abnormal muscle consistency and putting a unique pattern of tender points together. All of these requirements make the tender points objective findings.

6. Could the treatments of pain have caused the fibromyalgia, and not the original trauma?

ANSWER: Treatments of pain are intended to relieve the pain and improve the condition. Medical treatments for pain do not cause fibromyalgia, even though some of the medical treatments may not have helped to reduce the pain. The pain was caused from the original trauma, not from any medical treatments.

7. How can the condition persist years later when most healing occurs in six weeks?

ANSWER: Most healing will occur within six weeks, but not all injuries completely heal. Post-traumatic fibromyalgia is an example of a soft tissue condition that never heals but, rather, evolves into a chronic and permanent problem.

8. If you did not see the patient until over a year after the accident, how can you be certain a patient has post-traumatic fibromyalgia?

ANSWER: The ability to diagnose post-traumatic fibromyalgia does not depend on seeing the patient within a short time after the trauma. I believe post-traumatic fibromyalgia should not be diagnosed before six months following a trauma. The diagnosis depends on the complete clinical evaluation, including the patient history, the physical examination, review of previous available records and any diagnostic tests.

If the patient reports a history of chronic pain ever since a trauma, has characteristic painful tender points, and has no other medical conditions, I am able to put these pieces of the puzzle together and make a diagnosis of post-traumatic fibromyalgia with a reasonable degree of medical certainty, even if I haven't seen the patient for the first time until over a year after the accident.

9. Why didn't the emergency room doctor mention any pain or tender points at the time of his examination?

ANSWER: Painful tender points are not present immediately following a trauma. They take weeks to months to develop, so an emergency room doctor would not detect tender points during the emergency room evaluation unless the person has pre-existing fibromyalgia and pre-existing painful tender points.

It usually takes up to a few days for all of the injured areas to hurt; so it is not unusual for an area not to be painful at the time of the emergency room evaluation, but by the next day be extremely painful. It would not be unusual, therefore, for an emergency room doctor not to mention any pain and tender points in a particular region at the time of the examination immediately after the trauma.

10. Could stress have caused the fibromyalgia?

ANSWER: Stress is not considered a cause of fibromyalgia. Once an individual has fibromyalgia, stress is known to aggravate or cause a flare-up of fibromyalgia. Everyone experiences stress as a part of everyday life, but not everyone develops fibromyalgia. Even those who experience higher stress have not been shown to develop more fibromyalgia. Therefore, we cannot state that stress is a cause of fibromyalgia.

11. *If the individual had depression, irritable bowel syndrome and difficulty sleeping prior to the accident, did she not have fibromyalgia prior to the accident?*

ANSWER: All of these conditions are common. Just because an individual had one or more of these conditions prior to an accident does not mean the person had fibromyalgia prior to the accident. That is like putting the cart before the horse. One needs to have chronic pain and painful tender points in order to have a diagnosis of fibromyalgia. These are the key features to fibromyalgia, not whether associated conditions such as depression, irritable bowel syndrome or difficulty sleeping are present.

12. *Could this person be faking fibromyalgia?*

ANSWER: I do not think this person is faking fibromyalgia. I found the person to be truthful in her history and have no reason to believe she is being dishonest with me.

My physical exam has confirmed the presence of tender points in an objective pattern that could not be faked; so I conclude that this patient has post-traumatic fibromyalgia on the basis of my clinical evaluation and impression.

13. *Did you conclude that this person has post-traumatic fibromyalgia by reviewing the records even before you saw the patient?*

ANSWER: I never assume a person has any diagnosis before I even see the person. Whenever I first see a patient who has pain, I want to make sure that the pain is not from cancer or some other life-threatening condition. I may briefly review records that have been provided beforehand, but I rely on my own clinical evaluation including a complete history and physical examination to come up with my own diagnosis. My diagnosis is always reached after the clinical evaluation and never before.

14. **Are you an advocate for the patient with fibromyalgia?**

    ANSWER: I am a doctor who tries to help patients whether they have pain, weakness or other problems. I try to do my best to provide the highest degree of competent, compassionate care to my patients, regardless of their diagnosis.

15. **Are you being paid for this testimony?**

    ANSWER: I am being paid for my time involved in reviewing the chart and providing testimony.

15

The Future in Fibromyalgia

Physicians of all specialties are learning more about fibromyalgia and are becoming better at diagnosing this condition. Post-traumatic fibromyalgia is also becoming more recognized in the courts and industries, and the number of people who receive this diagnosis will increase as the result of this increased awareness. Post-traumatic fibromyalgia will continue to have significant social, economic and legal impacts on the individual and the community.

Much research is being carried out to help us get a better picture of fibromyalgia, including post-traumatic fibromyalgia. Various research areas include developing new medications and therapies that are more specific for controlling fibromyalgia symptoms and researching the muscles (particularly the tender points) to better understand the actual pathological mechanism involved. Researchers are attempting to identify individuals who are more prone to getting this condition and determining what preventive or long-term measures may be effective. Studies investigating the pathologic mechanisms of trauma and fibromyalgia need to be completed.

Changes will occur in the insurance, Worker's Compensation, disability and court systems on dealing with fibromyalgia. The medical challenge is not only to fully understand fibromyalgia but to minimize its impact on the individual and the community until a cure is found. The social and economic challenge is to recognize and provide reasonable, medically necessary treatment to individuals with fibromyalgia without overwhelming the resources, but also not depriving individuals of necessary treatments.

As a physician with fibromyalgia, I hope that the medicolegal future in fibromyalgia will enable an individual suffering from fibromyalgia to get help and achieve the highest level of function possible in the community.

Index

Q

R

S

T

More Ways for "Helping You Live Life to the Fullest"

If you enjoyed *Understanding Post-Traumatic Fibromyalgia*, you will be interested in other resources from Anadem Publishing. Anadem Publishing is devoted to providing health information to assist patients with chronic conditions in taking charge of their recovery and in getting the most out of life.

Fibromyalgia – Managing the Pain
by Mark Pellegrino, M.D.

Dr. Pellegrino delivers a comprehensive guide to the syndrome. It is the ideal book for the recently diagnosed FMS patient from the doctor whose treats fibromyalgia patients and has it himself.

The Fibromyalgia Survivor
by Mark Pellegrino, M.D.

The *Fibromyalgia Survivor* is packed with good advice and tips on every aspect of living your life to the fullest. You get the specific step-by-step "how to's" for daily living. Plus, you learn Fibronomics, the four key principles that help you minimize your pain in every situation.

The Fibromyalgia Supporter
by Mark Pellegrino, M.D.

How do you help loved ones really understand what they need to know about your fibromyalgia? Dr. Pellegrino explains to your loved ones how it feels, how they can become "supporters," and how you and your loved ones can still have a wonderful life together.

Laugh at Your Muscles
by Mark Pellegrino, M.D.
An easy, light read that you can enjoy and benefit from.

Chronic Fatigue Syndrome: Charting Your Course to Recovery
by Mary E. O'Brien, M.D.

Mary O'Brien, M.D., shares her personal experience in overcoming many of the debilitating effects of Chronic Fatigue Syndrome. In an easy-to-read, nontechnical format, Dr. O'Brien shares advice on treatment options and self-help steps that will help you rebuild your stamina.

TMJ – Its Many Faces
by Wesley Shankland, D.D.S., M.S.

Fibromyalgia patients frequently suffer from TMJ disorders and orofacial pain. Dr. Shankland's book is filled with step-by-step instructions on how to relieve TMJ, head, neck, and facial pain.

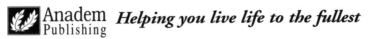 *Helping you live life to the fullest*

Order Your Books Today!

30 Day Money Back Guarantee
For fastest service, call 1•(800)•633•0055

Qty	Title	Price (US$)	Ohio Price*	Total
	Fibromyalgia: Managing the Pain	$12.45	$13.17	
	The Fibromyalgia Survivor	$19.50	$20.62	
	The Fibromyalgia Supporter	$15.50	$16.39	
	Understanding Post-Traumatic Fibromyalgia	$16.25	$17.18	
	TMJ – Its Many Faces	$19.50	$20.62	
	Laugh At Your Muscles	$ 5.95	$ 6.29	
	CFS – Charting Your Course to Recovery	$14.25	$15.07	

Shipping and handling

For 1 book, add $3.50

2–4 books, add $7.00

5-6 books, add $10.00

7+, please call

Priority mail, add $2.50

*Ohio price includes 5.75% state sales tax

Subtotal

Add Shipping and handling (see chart at left)

Total

☐ Enclosed is my check, made payable to Anadem, Inc.

☐ Charge my credit card: ☐ Master ☐ VISA

Card No. _____ **Exp.** _____

Signature _____

Name _____

Address _____

City _____ **State** ____ **Zip** _____ **Phone (** **)** _____

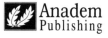

Anadem Publishing

3620 North High Street • Columbus, OH • 43214
1-800-633-0055 • FAX (614) 262-6630
http://www.anadem.com

You can count on Anadem Publishing to keep you informed of the newest, most advanced ideas to help you get the most out of life. Let us know if you want to be placed on our mailing list to be notified of new resources. And come visit us at our website! http://www.anadem.com